EAT THIS NOT THAT! 2012

11/11/21

The No-Diet Weight-Loss Solution
UK Edition

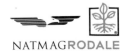

NATMAGRODALE

Editor-in-Chief Morgan Rees

Editor Tom Stone

Art Editor Paul Aarons

Editorial Assistant Thom Atkinson

Eat This, Not That! is a registered trademark of Rodale Inc.

© 2011 by Rodale Inc / Natmag-Rodale Ltd.

Cover Photography Studio 33

Interior Photography Studio 33 and Paul Aarons

With the exception of the following pages: page 47, 49, 51, 52, 53, 54, 55, 56, 57 59, 60, 223-239, 316 -319 Mitch Mandel and Thomas MacDonald/Rodale Images; 37, 39, 41, © Rodale Images; 68, 92, 112, 156, 180, 198, © Getty Images; 323-331 by mckibillo; 11-17 courtesy of all subjects

Based on the US edition by David Zinczenko with Matt Goulding.

Designed by George Karabotsos.

ISBN: 978–0–9568190–4–8

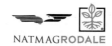

NATMAGRODALE

EAT THIS NOT THAT! 2012

DEDICATION

To all the men and women who care about health and who spread the word to friends and relatives about the importance of knowing what's really in our food. Because of your passionate efforts, food manufacturers and restaurant chains are waking up to the fact that more and more of us demand good, solid information about our food, and healthy choices that will help us drop pounds and stay lean for life.

And to the men and women working on the UK's farms and in supermarkets, as waiters and toiling in kitchens: it is because of your hard work that the British public have so many options. This book is designed to help us choose the best of what you've created.

The *ETNT* team

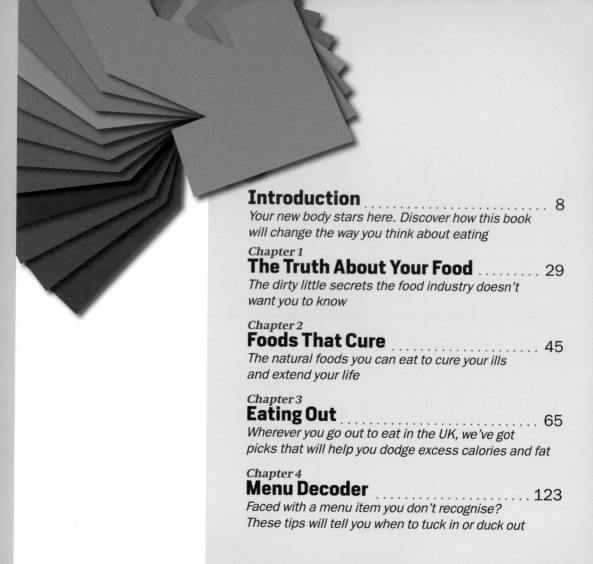

CONTENTS

Your new body is here.

It's here in these pages: that brand-new physique you've been waiting for; the leaner, fitter, healthier body you thought you'd never have. It's coming to you express delivery, without the need for dieting, for going hungry, for giving up anything *Eat This, Not That!* is ready to start stripping extra pounds from your body today. And once you lose that weight, you're going to keep it off. Forever.

I know what you're thinking: All that, just from a book? Won't I need something else, like a fancy home gym, a pricey personal trainer, a rice-cake-and-cottage-cheese diet, five hours a day of marathon training, a thousand pounds' worth of nutritional supplements, and an instruction manual that tells me how to turn my vacuum cleaner into a makeshift liposuction machine? No. Just this book.

That's because, *Eat This, Not That!* isn't a typical book. Yes, it's made of paper, with lots of photos and words. But the fact is, *Eat This, Not That!* is so revolutionary, so amazingly effective, you can lose weight without even reading it! Really? I don't have to read it? What do I do, rub it on my tummy?

Well, no: Of course we want you to read it—we worked hard on every word! And if you read it cover to cover, you'll discover it's packed with tonnes of information about the foods you eat that will shock and amaze you—and maybe even freak you out. But *Eat This, Not That!* wasn't created to be a sit-down-and-read-it type of book.

Eat This, Not That! is a tool

A peek-at-it-in-the-restaurant tool. A consult-it-in-the-supermarket tool. A whip-it-out-at-the-takeaway tool. A veritable Swiss Army knife of fat fighting, a weight-loss coach in your pocket. It's designed to make smart food choices easier, no matter where you're making them. And it just might be the best health-boosting, fat-fighting investment you'll ever make. Consider just a handful of real stories from real people who've shed 5 stone—or more!—of unwanted, unhealthy flab, using previous international editions of this book, and you'll understand why we call it "The no-diet weight-loss solution":

▶ **MICHAEL COLOMBO,** *shed 6.5 stone* in just over 8 months and conquered life-threatening sleep apnoea, after picking up a copy of *Eat This, Not That!* "My confidence has sky-rocketed!" he says. (Read his full story on the opposite page). And he never had to go on a diet or skip a meal!

▶ **ERIKA BOWEN,** *dropped 6 stone*—without dieting. "I feel like I've always wanted to feel," she says. Once she discovered the truth about her food, she learned she could lose weight and never feel hungry. (You'll find her true-life tale on page 13.)

▶ **DANA BICKELMAN,** *lost 5 stone* after discovering the shocking truth about the foods she was eating. Her secret: She learned to indulge—even at her favourite restaurants—but to do it more smartly. "Men want to say hello to me now, and that's great," she says. "I've never had this kind of attention before!" (Read her whole tale on page 15.)

Never dieting, never skipping meals, never going hungry? Always eating what you want, when you want, where you want? And still losing all the weight you want?

Think it sounds impossible? Like I'm trying to sell you some tartan paint or a tin of elbow grease?

Well, it's not impossible. In fact, it's scientifically proven. And here's why: Many of the foods we eat today—from common supermarket products to takeaway snacks to sit-down dinners at chain restaurants, and even some popular "health" foods—are far worse for our waistlines than we could ever imagine. That's because food companies have spent the past few generations devising ever more creative ways to pack our food with fat, salt, and sugar in an effort to hit the ultimate sweet spot on our palates, the bull's-eye on our

"I'm finally happy when I look in the mirror."

Michael Colombo, a long-time *Men's Health* magazine reader, had always been bigger than his mates. "I was always the type of person whom you'd describe as 'chunky,'" he says. "I liked to say I was big-boned." But it was when he moved out of his parents' house and began to live on his own that he grew much larger, and "big-boned" went form a wink-wink euphemism into a big form of denial.

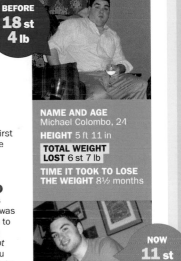

BEFORE
18 st 4 lb

NAME AND AGE
Michael Colombo, 24

HEIGHT 5 ft 11 in

TOTAL WEIGHT LOST 6 st 7 lb

TIME IT TOOK TO LOSE THE WEIGHT 8½ months

NOW
11 st 11 lb

THE "A-HA!" MOMENT

Even after Michael tipped the scales past 17 stone, he never considered himself obese. "I turned to food for pleasure and comfort, and my weight spiralled downhill to the point where I didn't even realise I'd become as heavy as I had," he says. His moment of motivation to lose weight came after a holiday with friends. "I saw pictures from after we got back, and I couldn't believe that was me, that I was that big." Those pictures were all it took—the same week he returned from the holiday, he joined a gym and bought his first *Eat This, Not That!* book, which he'd read about in *Men's Health*. "I decided this was going to be it, and I would turn my weight around, no matter how hard it was."

THE TURNING POINT

For the first 2 weeks of Michael's new routine, he refused to step on the scales. "I was afraid I wouldn't have lost much weight and I'd be discouraged and give up," he says. "But when I got on, I had lost 5 pounds—and that made such a difference in my motivation."

HIS NEW LIFE

Michael says he feels like a different person after having lost more than 6 stone. For starters, he's sleeping much better. "I used to have sleep apnea, and would wake up in the middle of the night. But now I sleep all the way through." He says he doesn't even snore anymore.

Even more impressive to Michael is the effect it's had on his self-esteem. "I'm finally happy when I look in the mirror," he says. "I have a lot more confidence to meet new people, because I'm not concerned with how I look, or how they'll perceive me when we're first introduced. My confidence has rocketed."

HOW *EAT THIS, NOT THAT!* HELPED

Before Michael began his new lifestyle, he says he was concerned that he'd have to starve himself in order to lose weight. "*Eat This, Not That!* showed me that you don't have to go completely crazy with your diet—it taught me that there are good options out there other than tiny salads or 'health food' fads."

He says that the section on drinks was a life-saver. "I have a sweet tooth, and I've always loved fizzy drinks and smoothies. But the list showed me that while companies might market smoothies as the healthier alternatives, they're often not."

"*Eat This, Not That! taught me that there are options out there other than tiny salads and 'health food' fads.*"

tongues. That's why so many of our foods now have ingredients that, when read aloud, sound like characters from a science-fiction novel—characters like Trans-Fatty Acid (sounds like a cross-dressing hippie, but in fact it's a cholesterol-promoting fat) and Soy Isolate (could be the name of a Chinese hermit, but is in fact a refined protein that may actually undermine testosterone). It's all part of an effort on the part of food manufacturers to make us rush out to buy more. But the unnatural foods they've created trigger unnatural hunger and unnatural cravings. And those unnatural cravings for unnatural foods lead to something else: unnatural weight gain. Today's food is far higher in fat, salt, sugar, and calories than the foods our grandparents ate. In fact, British children now spend more than twice the amount that American children do on unhealthy snacks like crisps and chocolate (£372 a year here, compared to just £150 a year in the United States), according to independent research company Datamonitor. No wonder we're in the throes of an obesity epidemic beyond the scope of anything humankind has ever seen. And look at what it's doing to our world:

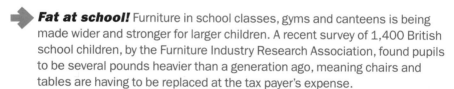

Fat at school! Furniture in school classes, gyms and canteens is being made wider and stronger for larger children. A recent survey of 1,400 British school children, by the Furniture Industry Research Association, found pupils to be several pounds heavier than a generation ago, meaning chairs and tables are having to be replaced at the tax payer's expense.

Fat on the NHS! Currently the direct cost of obesity to the NHS is estimated to be around £4.2 billion. This is forecast to more than double by 2050 if obesity levels go unchecked. This money is used for general care of overweight individuals, who are liable to suffer from a range of related disorders, such as type 2 diabetes. More controversially it's also used to pay for drastic solutions to obesity such as weight-loss surgery (gastric bands and bypasses). One British family of three who hit the headlines recently have all undergone gastric surgery, along with a range of other treatment, which in total is estimated to have cost the tax payer £1.2 million.

"I needed a way to make this weight loss last."

Growing up, **Erika Bowen** had been athletic—she played volleyball and ran for her school, and barely ever thought about her weight. She began to gain more at University, but even then didn't consider herself fat. "Even when I hit 14 stone, I didn't think it was such a big deal," she says.

THE "A-HA!" MOMENT

In reality, though, Erika's weight was affecting several aspects of her life. She began to have to shop online, because the high street no longer carried clothing in her size. And when she turned 27, she and her husband started trying to have a baby—and were unsuccessful. "There wasn't any real medical reason for why we couldn't get pregnant, but one theory was that I needed to get my weight under control. My BMI was 40, and the doctors said that might affect successful conception."

Just two weeks before she turned 29, she went to the doctor for a checkup and learned that she weighed 17 stone 12 pounds. "That was a huge eye-opener for me. I thought: Oh my God, I've wasted my 20s. So that's when I decided I had to do something."

THE TURNING POINT

After losing 6 pounds with the help of a trainer, Erika bought the first edition of *Eat This, Not That!* Once she began incorporating healthy eating with exercise, she saw the weight start to melt off. "My original goal was to lose 3.5 stone," she says. Six stone later, she's 10 pounds away from her goal weight: 155 pounds.

The most notable point for her, she says, is the first time she ran outside. "When I first ran outside, I realised, I'm one of those people. But now I look forward to my run with my dog every day. "

HER NEW LIFE

"There was a time when I refused to wear tank tops," she says. "But now I'm very comfortable in my own skin, and I'm wearing things I'd never have worn before." Her husband has told her she acts like a happier person now, and her friends leave ego-boosting comments on her Facebook wall. "They tell me my out ward appearance now reflects my inner beauty," she says. "I feel like I've always wanted to feel. Other people are finally seeing me the way I've always seen myself."

HOW *EAT THIS, NOT THAT!* HELPED

"I knew I couldn't do Atkins or South Beach or Weight Watchers, because I like to be in control of things—I want to eat what I want to eat," Erika says. The concept of *Eat This, Not That!* appealed to her because of the freedom it allowed. "I love crisps. And this book has taught me that I don't have to give them up."

"I need a way to make this weight loss last. It might have come off quicker, but I wouldn't have maintained it as much as I have. *Eat This, Not That!* is more about lifestyle."

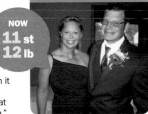

BEFORE
17 st
12 lb

NAME AND AGE
Erika Bowen, 30
HEIGHT 5 ft 7 in
TOTAL WEIGHT LOST 6 st
TIME IT TOOK TO LOSE THE WEIGHT 17 months

NOW
11 st
12 lb

"Other people are finally seeing me the way I've always seen myself."

13

Fat in hospital! Hospitals across the land are having to strengthen or completely replace beds in order to safely accommodate larger patients. Sunderland Royal Hospital recently revealed it was spending £300,000 on special beds, including four for the morbidly obese and 152 for heavier-than-normal patients.

Fat enough to call the fire brigade! An increasing problem for the fire service is being called out, not to put out fires, but to winch "excessively overweight" people out of situations where they have become stuck in "beds, baths or chairs." The NHS says that these people have essentially become "too fat to walk". While this is the extreme end of our nation's weight problem, there were still over 128 of these types of emergency in the second half of the last decade, costing over £300,000. This figure is certain to balloon by the end of this decade.

Fat enough to hurt the economy! The government estimates that, quite apart from the direct burden placed on NHS services by the nation's weight problem, the indirect cost to the wider economy could be as much as £16 billion, due to issues such as reduced worker productivity and sickness.

Fat from the cradle to the grave! Local authorities are having to spend money widening crematoria furnaces to accommodate bigger bodies in bigger coffins. The new Bishop Auckland crematorium in the Wear Valley can take coffins up to 43 inches wide – 13 inches more than the conventional 30 inch coffin.

In fact, we're now eating so much, and getting so fat, that we don't even recognise ourselves as overweight. One study in the *British Medical Journal* found that in Great Britain the size at which we perceive ourselves to be overweight has risen significantly. Researchers conducted two surveys of over 1,500 people. They discovered that in 1999 81% of overweight participants correctly identified their weight problem. By 2007 this had fallen to 75%,

"I've never had this kind of attention before."

Dana Bickelman says that she'd been overweight her entire life. "I always used food in reaction to every emotion, whether it was a good moment or a bad." She thought she'd tried every method of losing weight—Weight Watchers, boot camps, gym memberships—but nothing stuck. "Food used to control my life," she says. "I'd eat and eat and then feel terrible about it afterwards." It was a spiral that she thought she'd never come out of.

THE "A-HA!" MOMENT

Dana saw the first edition of *Eat This, Not That!* on a shelf and bought it impulsively. But the concept appealed to her, she says, because it wasn't as strict as a regular diet plan. "I don't like someone telling me how I should diet, exactly how much I should eat. *Eat This, Not That!* offered useful tips, rather than a strict plan."

She was shocked to learn how many calories were in foods she ate regularly. "Once I started being more aware of what I was eating, the weight started coming off."

THE TURNING POINT

Eat This, Not That! taught Dana how to read food labels. "I learned all about portion control, and that so many packaged foods have a ton of added sugar and additives." Once she finally understood what she was putting into her body, she says she started losing weight more quickly.

Portion control was also key. "I was eating this small serving size of ice cream, and I realised I was content with eating half of it. The idea that I didn't have to eat the whole thing was shocking, and made me feel so much more in control."

HER NEW LIFE

Everything in Dana's life has been affected by her weight loss. She's become better at her job: As a case manager for people with disabilities, she's brought the knowledge gained from *Eat This, Not That!* to her work, and teaches her clients how to read product labels and shop smarter. "Nutrition is something I'm really passionate about now, and I really want to help people learn about it."

And her self-esteem is the highest it's ever been.

"Men want to say hi to me now, and that's great. I've never had this kind of attention before. It's wonderful."

HOW *EAT THIS, NOT THAT!* HELPED

Dana brings the book to her favourite restaurants. "It's so great that I can still eat there and enjoy the food, but know that I'm not overdoing it."

She says she incorporates the tips into her lifestyle, and feels confident that she's making smart food decisions along the way. "*Eat This, Not That!* has changed my life. I bring the books with my colleagues into the supermarket, and we'll go around and read labels, and they're shocked. It's not just one type of person who's going to benefit from this type of stuff; it's everyone."

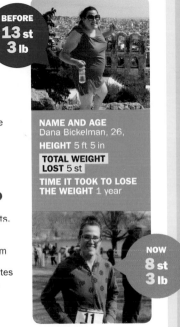

BEFORE 13 st 3 lb

NAME AND AGE
Dana Bickelman, 26,

HEIGHT 5 ft 5 in

TOTAL WEIGHT LOST 5 st

TIME IT TOOK TO LOSE THE WEIGHT 1 year

NOW 8 st 3 lb

"It's not just one type of person who's going to benefit from this type of stuff; it's everyone."

demonstrating a decrease in the sensitivity of self diagnosis. Or, to put it another way, we're so used to being surrounded by fat—our own and others'—that we no longer recognise it as fat.

Now consider what this is costing us: In 2006, the army raised the Body Mass Index acceptable for new recruits from 28 to 32—to within the 'obese' range. This was after the Nation Audit Office revealed that only a third of all 16 year olds met the old target. Now it would appear the policy has backfired as leaked internal documents from the Ministry of Defence reported that in 2010, up to two thirds of soldiers were unfit for combat

Those are some overwhelming, and terrifying, numbers. But why is this happening? Is it all because we've suddenly become gluttons with nothing on our minds but eating and eating and eating some more?

No. It's because food companies have come up with ever more sneaky ways to get us to buy more and more of their products. And there's little protection for consumers, and not nearly enough information out there to help us make smart choices.

Take the supermarket: Despite regulations that force packaged-foods manufacturers to print nutritional information on most of their goods, hijinks persist. Here's a great example: next time you're in the dairy section take a look at Yeo Valley Organic Fat Free Vanilla Yogurt—sounds healthy doesn't it? But that's until you realise that a serving packs 21 grams of sugar—more than a Cadbury's Flake. *Eat This, Not That!* will tip you off to these food tricks and help make the right choice easy.

It gets even dicier in restaurant chains, many of which still refuse to make nutritional information available to their customers. So *Eat This, Not That!* has gone behind the scenes, using food labs to uncover hidden calorie counts, and make smart eating easier than ever.

"I look at pictures and can't believe I'm the same person."

As a computer programmer, **Jeff Small's** life was dominated by long, sedentary hours sitting in front of a computer screen. "I stayed up late, I ate fast food all the time, and I ate at all hours of the night," he says. And not because he didn't know better, but rather out of sheer lack of motivation to live more healthily. "I knew the lifestyle I was leading wasn't a recipe for health, but I didn't know how soon it would come back to haunt me."

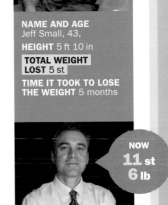

BEFORE
16 st 6 lb

NAME AND AGE
Jeff Small, 43,

HEIGHT 5 ft 10 in

TOTAL WEIGHT LOST 5 st

TIME IT TOOK TO LOSE THE WEIGHT 5 months

NOW
11 st 6 lb

THE "A-HA!" MOMENT

A routine doctor visit around Christmas 2008 revealed a few scary facts: He weighed 16 stone 6 pounds. His blood pressure and bad cholesterol were through the roof. The doctor told him that if he didn't get his weight in check, he was at high risk for heart disease and stroke.

He began by setting up an exercise bike in his garage, and he rode incrementally farther and harder each day. Soon Jeff realized: "I need to start putting better food into my body, too."

THE TURNING POINT

"The *Eat This, Not That!* supermarket section helped me to take control of my life," he says. "It arms you with the ability to walk into a supermarket and know that you made the right decisions about the food you are going to eat for the entire week." By

May, he had lost 5 stone, and friends weren't even recognising him when they passed him on the street.

HIS NEW LIFE

"I'm a completely different person in my job. It changed how people interacted with me at work, it changed how people wanted to invite me to meetings, and it even changed the way I participated in those meetings."

The weight loss also impacted his marriage. "I had low self-esteem and low energy, and I never wanted to go out and do things. I didn't feel that my wife found me attractive." But after the transformation, he says, all those problems disappeared. "I look at pictures of myself from before and I can't believe I'm the same person."

HOW *EAT THIS, NOT THAT!* HELPED

He learned to eat small snacks throughout the day to keep from getting hungry and over-indulging during meals. "People ask me how I stay so fit when I eat so much, and I tell them it's because I'm always eating that I can keep the weight off. I eat smart things every 2 to 3 hours, and I'm never hungry."

Jeff also loves the Cook This, Not That! chapter: "I love to cook, and the recipes are delicious."

FINAL THOUGHTS:

"I'm 43 years old and nothing has ever changed my life as much as *Eat This, Not That!* Nothing has had such an impact on my life as that book because it allowed me to shop the way I shop and eat the way I eat."

"Nothing has ever had as big an impact on my life as this book."

★ *Let's say you're out shopping.* You pass by a branch of Eat and be tempted by the delicious coffee smells and decide to pop in for a caffeine fix and a sandwich. The choice you make at the counter could have a big effect on your waistline. Do you fancy a cheese and pickle sandwich or a beef and horseradish? Would you like a flat white or a chai latte? Opt for the seemingly innocent cheese and pickle with the latte on the side and you'll ingest 546 extra calories – almost a third of your recommended daily amount! (Make that wrong choice just twice a month and you'll pack an additional 4 pounds of fat onto your body in a year!)

★ *Or maybe you stop at the petrol station to fill up your tank as well as your car's.* You might decide to plug a gap with an indulgent two Curly Wurlys or go for a Boost Bar. But make the wrong selection and you'll be wolfing down an extra 80 calories and more than twice the saturated fat. (Hint: sometimes less is more.)

★ *Or, you're in the supermarket trying to buy the right stuff, and you grab Eat Natural Gluten Free Toasted Muesli With Buckwheat to eat for your breakfast in the coming week.* It's "natural," for heaven's sake, and that buckwheat's got to be healthy, right? But if you had gone for Alpen No Added Sugar, you'd be saving 90 calories and 9g of fat every time you pour a bowl. That's 630 calories per week!

By making smart food swaps, you can cut hundreds, even thousands, of calories out of your food intake every day, and still enjoy the treat at the shops, the snack at the petrol station, or lunch, dinner, or breakfast at your favourite restaurant. As we've seen above, it's not just a matter of how you look; it's a matter of health, of well-being—it's even a matter of national security!

Smart swaps equal fewer calories. Fewer calories equal fewer pounds and a longer, healthier, happier life. It's as simple as that.

How you can use this book to make losing weight easy

If you want to shed belly fat, there's only one formula you need to know, and luckily for you, it's easier than anything you encountered in algebra at school.

The magic formula is this
Calories in − calories out = total weight loss or gain. This is the equation that determines whether your body will shape up to look more like a slender 1 or a paunchy 0, a flat-bellied metre-stick or a pot-bellied protractor. That's why it's absolutely critical that you understand the numbers you're plugging into this formula.

On the "calories out" side, we have your daily activities: cleaning house, standing in line at the post office, hauling in groceries, and so on. Often when people discover extra flab hanging around their midsections, they assume there's something wrong with this side of the equation. Maybe so, but more likely it's the front-end of the equation—the "calories in" side—that's tipping the scale. That side keeps track of all the biscuits, fried chicken, and piles of pasta that you eat every day.

In order to maintain a healthy body weight, a moderately active woman between the ages of 20 and 50 needs 2,000 to 2,200 calories per day. A man

fitting the same profile needs 2,400 to 2,600. Those numbers can fluctuate depending on whether you're taller or shorter than average or whether you spend more or less time exercising, but they represent reasonable estimations for most people. (For a more accurate assessment, use the calorie calculator at mayoclinic.com)

Let's take a closer look at the numbers It takes 3,500 calories to create a pound of body fat. So if you eat an extra 500 per day—just 10 calories more than the amount in a Big Mac—then you'll earn 1 new pound of body fat each week. Make that a habit—like so many of us do unwittingly—and you'll gain 3 stone and 10 pounds of flab per year!

That's where this book comes in. Within these pages are literally hundreds of simple food swaps that will save you from 10 to 1,000 calories or more apiece. The more often you choose "Eat This" foods over "Not That!" options, the quicker you'll notice layers of fat disappearing from your body. Check this out:

• A single bowl of **SPECIAL K HONEY CLUSTERS** cereal has 175 calories. Switch to **CRUNCHY NUT CORNFLAKES** five

times per week and you'll drop 4 pounds this year.

• A **GRANDE COFFEE FRAPPUCCINO** from Starbucks has 241 calories. Switch to a **SEMI-SKIMMED ICED CAFFE LATTE** three times per week and you'll shed 2½ pounds in 6 months.

• **TESCO FINEST SPAGHETTI CARBONARA** has 890 calories. Make the switch to their **LIGHT CHOICES HAM AND MUSHROOM TAGLIATELLE** three times per week and you'll drop an extra 5½ pounds every 3 months.

• A **CAFE ROUGE SALADE PAYSANNE** packs in an astounding 1,101 calories. Instead, order their **SALADE CAESAR** (529) three times per week—or make a comparative swap at some other restaurant—and you'll blast away more than 4 pounds of body fat in just 2 months.

And here's the best news of all: These swaps aren't isolated calorie savers. If you commit yourself to just the four on this list, the cumulative calorie-saving effect will eliminate over a pound of body fat every week this year. Take that, multigrain bagel! Check out eight more of our favourite calorie-squashing, fat-melting Top Swaps on the following pages.

Burgers

Save!
244 calories
and
19 g fat!

Eat This!
McDonald's Big Mac

490 calories
24 g fat
(10 g saturated)
2.1 g salt

Not That!
Burger King Whopper
with Cheese

734 calories
43 g fat
(13 g saturated)
3.7 g salt

In the battle of the burgers McDonald's comes out on top. The Big Mac adds flavour with healthy gherkins, compared to the Whopper, which is loaded up with calorific mayonnaise. You get cheese as standard on the double-stacked Big Mac, but with Burger King's signature sandwich you have to order it separately and when you do you add 83 calories and 7 grams of fat to a burger that already has plenty of both. If you're a Whopper addict resist the cheese and ask for it to be made without mayo and you'll get the calories down below the 600 mark... but it might be tastier to go to McDonald's, especially when you consider that you'll be saving a quarter of your guideline daily amount of salt.

Pasta

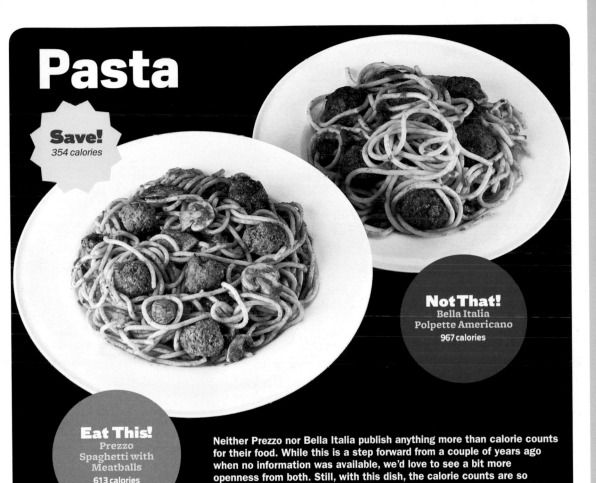

Save!
354 calories

Not That!
Bella Italia
Polpette Americano
967 calories

Eat This!
Prezzo
Spaghetti with
Meatballs
613 calories

Neither Prezzo nor Bella Italia publish anything more than calorie counts for their food. While this is a step forward from a couple of years ago when no information was available, we'd love to see a bit more openness from both. Still, with this dish, the calorie counts are so dramatically different, the decision is easy. Bella Italia serves up thick, chunky spaghetti and oversized meatballs, that must pack a hefty fat punch. Prezzo, on the other hand offers lighter pasta, and meatballs that have a hand-made rather than a ready made feel.

Steak

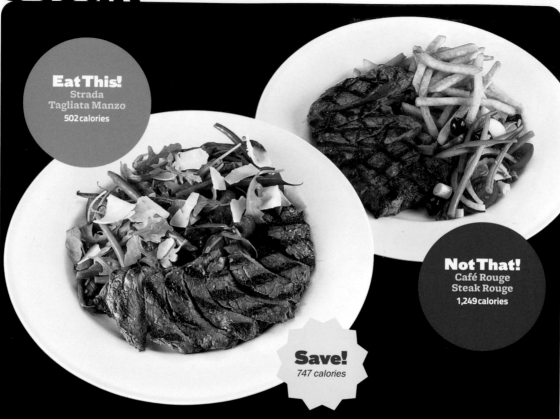

Eat This!
Strada
Tagliata Manzo
502 calories

Not That!
Café Rouge
Steak Rouge
1,249 calories

Save!
747 calories

Again, we'd love these two chains to publish more than just calories, but the difference here is so stark the healthier option is clear. Café Rogue don't hold back with their cut of steak or the sides. Those fries are loaded with fat and help to push the calorie count up. Strada do things differently. Sirloin is one of the leanest cuts and they go out on a limb by not serving it with chips. It might require a leap of faith, but the salad, with plenty of green beans and shavings of Parmesan is substantial enough to ensure you don't feel short changed. You can have a glass of wine with your meal and still walk away with a substantial calorie saving.

Sandwiches

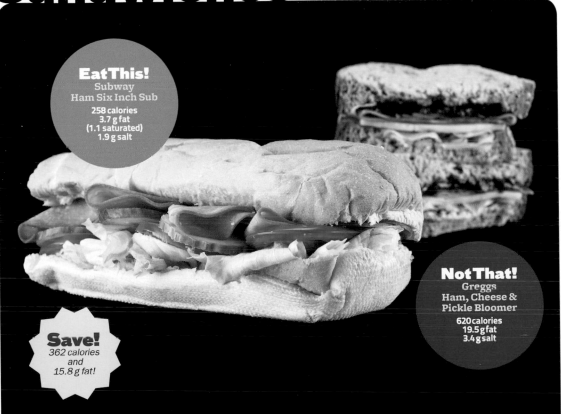

Eat This!
Subway
Ham Six Inch Sub

258 calories
3.7 g fat
(1.1 saturated)
1.9 g salt

Not That!
Greggs
Ham, Cheese &
Pickle Bloomer

620 calories
19.5 g fat
3.4 g salt

Save!
362 calories
and
15.8 g fat!

Greggs' innocent looking bloomer loses out in quite a big way to Subway's packed sub. Greggs seem to have gone to quite a lot of trouble to provide nutritional information on their website, but inexplicably leave out two of the most important entries – saturated fat and sugars. Nevertheless we can be pretty sure that a hefty chunk of the calories in this bloomer come from sugar in the pickle and that a reasonable proportion of that fat will be saturated from the cheese and ham. Take a trip to Subway for a lunch that will fill you up, and give you a complete breakdown as to exactly why.

Chicken

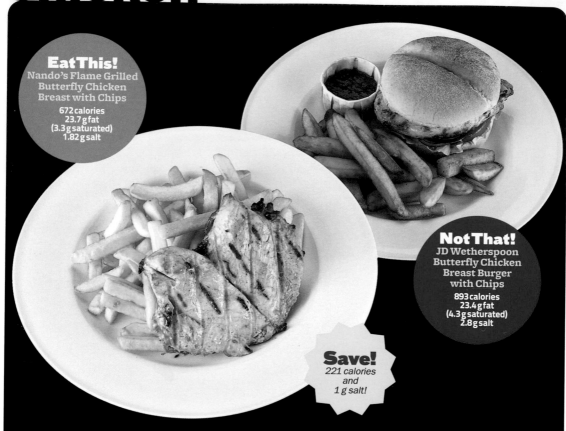

Eat This!
Nando's Flame Grilled
Butterfly Chicken
Breast with Chips

672 calories
23.7 g fat
(3.3 g saturated)
1.82 g salt

Not That!
JD Wetherspoon
Butterfly Chicken
Breast Burger
with Chips

893 calories
23.4 g fat
(4.3 g saturated)
2.8 g salt

Save!
221 calories
and
1 g salt!

Wetherspoon are at least attempting to clean up their act by offering this chicken burger on their menu which doesn't have a breaded coating (after all, who needs it when it's already served between two bits of bread?) But they are still pipped at the post by Portuguese giant Nando's, who add flavour to their chicken with their legendary peri peri coating (whereas Wetherspoon rely on calorific tomato relish) and chuck the bread out entirely. Also, thanks to the quality of their chicken breast, Nando's manage to cut saturated fat and salt levels, while getting more chips onto your plate. It's a win win.

Fruit Drinks

Drink This!
Caffè Nero:
Strawberry &
Raspberry Fruit
Booster

206 calories
1.5 g fat
44.6 g sugar

Save!
121 calories
and
10.3 g sugar!

Blindfolded you'd be hard pushed to taste the difference between these two fruit drinks. Both are icy, refreshing and packed with juicy berries. However, Costa manage to get an extra 10 grams of sugar into their version (that's as much as you get in two chocolate digestive biscuits). The calorie difference means that by the time you've sucked up the last of it you could have had half a pint of Guinness and a handful of nuts.

Not That!
Costa Red Berry
Fruit Cooler

327 calories
0.5 g fat
54.9 g sugar

Pizza

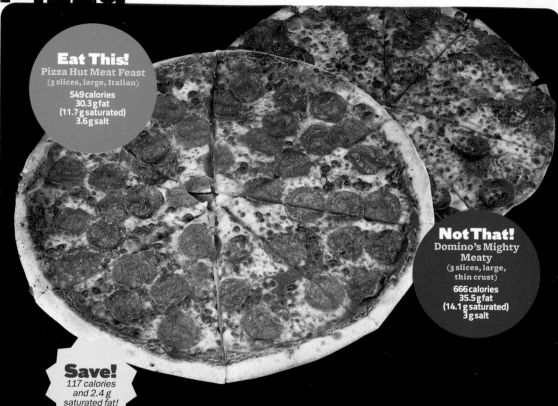

Eat This!
Pizza Hut Meat Feast
(3 slices, large, Italian)

549 calories
30.3 g fat
(11.7 g saturated)
3.6 g salt

Not That!
Domino's Mighty Meaty
(3 slices, large, thin crust)

666 calories
35.5 g fat
(14.1 g saturated)
3 g salt

Save!
117 calories
and 2.4 g
saturated fat!

These two pizzas are virtually identical, but Pizza Hut will save you over 100 calories over three slices. You might suspect that this is because Domino's must have more meat on their pizza, so some of those extra calories come from healthy protein. However, a quick glance at the toppings would suggest not and, more scientifically, the figures reveal you'll get an extra gram and a half of protein in each slice of the Pizza Hut version. In fact the only explanation for the higher calorie count at Domino's is the higher fat content, go to the Hut and you'll also save 10% of your guideline daily allowance for saturated fat.

Dessert

Save!
206 calories

Not That!
Pizza Express
Tiramisu
539 calories

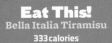

Eat This!
Bella Italia Tiramisu
333 calories

Both of these chains are shy about publishing more than calorie counts in their nutritional information. Nevertheless it's clear that the Pizza Express version of this Italian favourite is creamy, heavy and packed full of calories. Bella Italia's is a better bet. While it's never going to be a health food, the portion is slightly smaller and it's also lighter and fluffier, so a lot less trouble for your waistline. If you know you're going to want this dessert head to Bella Italia to indulge (and turn to our restaurant section from page 68 for other healthy options for the rest of your meal there).

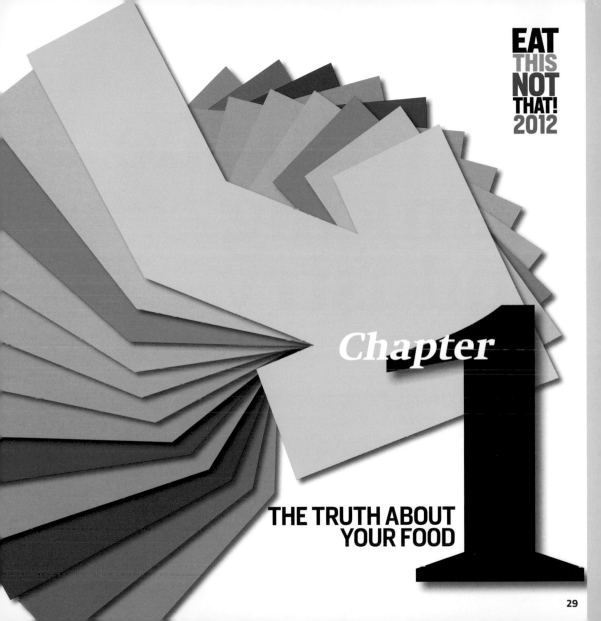

Chapter

1

THE TRUTH ABOUT YOUR FOOD

As with the banking industry,

the Russian political system, and the romantic liaisons in *Coronation Street*, all is not as it seems in the world of food and drink.

Misnomers and confusing labels have been with us for generations—at least since our hungry ancestors devoured the first hamburger (with no actual ham in it) and gobbled down the first hot dog (with no actual dog in it). And how many fried chicken shops in your area claim to be "world famous" or "the best"? (Wouldn't you think being so good might allow them to upgrade to some cleaner signs and menus?)

What a food seller chooses to call his product or how he chooses to advertise it has always been as much a matter of fiction and marketing as anything else. And everybody's in on the joke. Nobody believes that the man from Del Monte is really touring the world personally testing every fruit crop. Or that Aunt Bessie is slaving over a hot Aga in her country kitchen to bring you her famous

Yorkshire puddings. Or that there's a salty, bearded captain with a crew of happy children overseeing the day's catch of fish for Bird's Eye. These silly marketing claims and characters are just part of the commercial spin of modern life, and if they make one box of frozen fish sticks look somehow more appealing than the next, so be it.

But the hype and the spin get a little more serious—and a lot more unfair—when food starts to carry words that make one food seem "healthier" than another. Words and phrases like "lower in fat" or "all natural" or "multigrain" sound very appealing. Who wouldn't choose the all-natural multigrain product that's lower in fat?

The problem is, none of these words and phrases really mean anything. The food that's "lower in fat" simply has less fat than the original version of the product—the "lower in fat" version is probably still bulging with unnecessary calories. (And as you'll learn in the coming chapters, the type of fat you're eating matters more than the amount.) "All natural"? So are crude oil, snake venom, and botulism, but I wouldn't want to pay to eat any of those. And "multigrain" means nothing more than "made from more than one grain"—it sounds healthy, but if all those many grains have been stripped of their fibre and nutrients, you might as well be eating a teaspoon of pure sugar.

And therein lies the rub—and the reason for this book.

While the government has made some significant strides in getting nutritional information to the public—like requiring food packaging to carry nutrition labels—there's still so much room for obfuscation and outright mendacity that knowing what's in our food is never a certainty.

Why Food is Different Today

One in four British adults are now obese. How is this possible? You might say it's because we've all stopped exercising—except, there's a Fitness First or a Virgin Active in every town in the country and a JD Sports on every high street. You might say it's because we stopped watching what we eat—except that on any given week, half of the best-sellers on Amazon are diet or cookbooks. You might say it's because we all just stopped caring—except that liposuction and gastric band surgery are endemic. And you know and I know that the two most common phrases in the English lexicon are "I'm trying to watch my weight" and "Does this make me look fat?"

Unfortunately, a recent report by the EU bestowed upon Britain the honour of the fattest nation in Europe. The information released by the European Commission has shown that 23.9 percent of British women are obese, the highest rate in Europe. British male's came in second place with 22 percent of the population classed as obese—losing out to Malta who hold the highest male obesity rate—but taking the European obesity crown overall. So what's causing all this weight gain? Did all our stomachs get larger or our mouths expand? Of course not. We haven't changed. The food has changed.

▶ **WE'RE SUPERSIZING OUR LIVES.** Of course we want to be smart with our money, especially in tough times. So of course when we see the word "value," especially as it pertains to a "meal," we're going to want to go for it. Supersizing it at your local fast-food restaurant gives you an average of 73 per cent more calories for a mere 17 percent more in cost. Sounds like a bargain, until you realise that you don't need the 73 percent more calories!

▶ **WE'RE EATING THINGS OUR BODIES AREN'T SUPPOSED TO EAT.**
A generation ago, it was hard for manufacturers to create baked goods that would last. Most require oils, and oil runs and leaks at room temperature. But since the 1960s, manufacturers have been baking with—and restaurants have been frying with—something called "trans fat." Trans fat is cheap and effective: It makes crisps crispier and biscuits tastier; and it lets cooks fry pound after pound of chips without smoking up their kitchens. But trans fat has been shown to have a horrific effect on our bodies: It raises our LDL (bad) cholesterol, lowers our HDL (good) cholesterol, and increases our risk of heart disease and obesity. (If you see the words "partially hydrogenated" on the list of ingredients, it's trans fat.)

▶ **WE'RE CONSUMING WAY TOO MUCH HIDDEN SUGAR.** While we are actually buying less sugar in bags and putting less in our tea, a recent report found that over the last 30 years food manufacturers have doubled the amount of sugar they add to products. The sweet stuff is linked to obesity, bad teeth, diabetes, accelerated ageing and heart disease. Researchers from the University of Cambridge found that obese people dramatically underestimate the amount of sugar they consume each day. Some consumed as much as 207 grams, which is nearly 52 spoonfuls and four times the guideline daily amount. And most of it is hidden in everyday foods.

The result of all this manipulation is that we absorb more calories than would have been humanly possible a few decades ago. Our food and drink are so calorie-dense that it's hard to eat healthily. And the way that foods are sold, in shops and restaurants, has made smart nutritional choices harder and harder to make.

That's why *Eat This, Not That!* is such an invaluable resource for those who want to eat their favourite foods and not be ambushed by hidden fat, sugar, and calories.

The ETNT! Encyclopedia

UNPACKING THE MOST MISLEADING CLAIMS OF THE FOOD INDUSTRY

GOOD SOURCE OF...

It means that the product contains between 10 and 19 percent of your daily requirement for the mentioned nutrient. In other words, you would still have to eat between 5 and 10 servings to get your full day's value.

LOW FAT

To make this triumphant claim foodstuffs must contain no more than 3g of fat per 100g (though milk has a scale of its own). Sounds great. Problem is, that reduction in fat often comes with an increase in sugar and salt and, ultimately, no net nutritional gain to speak of.

MULTIGRAIN

This simply means that more than one type of grain was used in processing (e.g., wheat, rye, barley, rice). It doesn't, however, make any claim about the degree of processing used on those grains. The only trustworthy claim for whole grains is "100 percent wholemeal."

LIGHTLY BREADED

The phrase restaurants often use to distract diners from the fact that the food they're about to eat has been rolled in flour, egg, and bread crumbs and let loose in a vat of bubbling fat. It doesn't matter how light the breading is; it's the oil part that will get you.

COMPLIMENTARY

Usually seen with one of the following words: chips, bread, desserts, refills. In any case, the act of giving away low-cost, high-calorie foods is a common tactic restaurants use to add value to the "customer experience." Remember, just because it's free doesn't mean it won't cost you in calories.

POLYUNSATURATED FATS AND MONOUNSATURATED FATS

Spot the difference. Polyunsaturated fat (you'll find in sunflowers) has been proven to lower blood cholesterol levels, which may help to reduce the risk of heart disease. Monounsaturated fat (that's your olives) has been shown to do the same, just not as well. And saturated fat (butter, lard, etc) is the one to avoid whenever possible as it heightens cholesterol and contributes to serious heart problems.

SUPPORTS THE IMMUNE SYSTEM / HELPS MAINTAIN A HEALTHY HEART

We've heard these before, but where is the science? Luckily rules are in place to prevent misleading claims about specific health claims on packaging. Though watch out for general claims to overall good health such as "healthy option" on a menu with no nutritional values to support it.

LIGHT OR *LITE*

To be able to splash this ambiguous spelling across packaging it must be at least 30% lower in one of the typical values than a standard product. However, there's no telling what's in the original, meaning products such as Pizza Express House Light Dressing still pack nearly 25 percent of your day's saturated fat, per 100 millilitres.

HIGH FIBRE

These products must be at least 6g of fibre per 100g, but cereals such as Kellogg's Fruit 'n Fibre, although high in fibre, contain a good dose more sugar, fat and therefore calories than a bowl of Bran Flakes. Turn to our supermarket guide (p150) for more details on these misnomers.

The Truth about Your Food

Just as the titans of the restaurant industry seek to obscure the reality behind their most dubious products and practices, so packaged goods aren't always quite what they seem. What does that mean to you? It means you're spending your hard-earned cash and calories on foods you may be undermining your health in ways you never even considered. Eating well is hard enough, but when companies start complicating matters with ambiguous label claims, that's when you need to arm yourself with the latest science and a few simple, savvy methods for outsmarting the food powers that be. What follows is just that, an insight into the most misunderstood foods in the UK, that will help you separate fact from fiction in a quest to getting exactly what you bargained for every time you go to the supermarket.

The truth about...
DIET FIZZY DRINKS

When confronted with the growing tide of calories from sweetened beverages, the first response is, "Why not just buy a diet drink?" Well, there are plenty of reasons why not.

Just because "light" versions are low in calories doesn't mean they can't lead to weight gain. Your favourite can of diet drink may have only five or fewer calories, but emerging research suggests that consuming sugary-tasting beverages—even if they're artificially sweetened—may lead to a greater preference for sweetness overall. That means you'll tend towards sweeter (and more calorific) cereal, bread, dessert—everything. Whatever the reason, it's clear that people who drink a lot of diet soft drinks aren't doing themselves any favours. New research from the University of Texas Health Science Centre found that people who drink diet on a daily basis have an increased risk of developing type 2 diabetes and metabolic syndrome. To top it all off drinking diet will mean

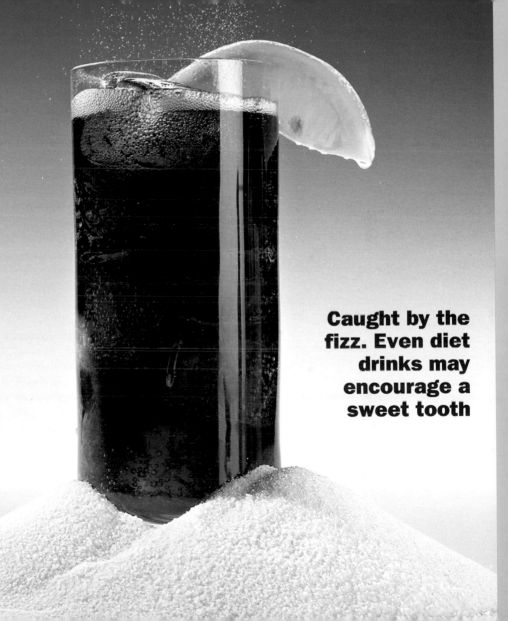

Caught by the fizz. Even diet drinks may encourage a sweet tooth

you're less inclined to go for the good stuff. In other words the more soft drinks you consume, the less thirsty you'll be, so the less you'll feel like having healthy beverages, like water and tea. This can ultimately hinder your health.

The truth about...
FREE-RANGE MEAT & EGGS
The claim sounds idyllic enough to reassure even the most ethical omnivore. But this popular buzzword might not live up to the peaceful, rolling-hills freedom it evokes.

Technically, free-range chickens must have access to the outdoors for at least eight hours each day. However, European Union free-range regulations require only that the land be "mainly covered with vegetation", without specifying the variety of plant or the condition they may be in. So the term could mean anything from a field to a puny pen. Products with free-range certificates have only meet the minimum legislative requirements. Though it can mean any number of things, free-range is certainly an improvement on food that doesn't bear the label at all. But for the best reared animals of all you should look for both free range and organic labels. That means you can be sure the animal hasn't been exposed to any chemicals. Plus organic certification carries with his more stringent general rules about how animals are kept.

The truth about...
FRUIT-IN-THE-CORNER YOGURTS
It seems like the ideal breakfast or snack for a man or woman on the go— a perfect combination of yogurt and antioxidant-packed fruits, pulled together in one convenient little cup. But are they really good for you?

While the yogurt offers stomach-soothing live cultures and a decent serving of protein, the sugar content of these seemingly healthy products is sky-high. The fruit itself is swimming in thick syrup—so much of it, in fact, that sugar (and other such sweeteners) often shows up on the ingredients list well before the fruit itself. And these low-quality refined carbohydrates are the last thing you want for breakfast— Australian researchers found that people whose diets were high in carbohydrates had lower metabolism than those who ate proportionally more protein. Not to mention, spikes in your blood sugar can wreck your

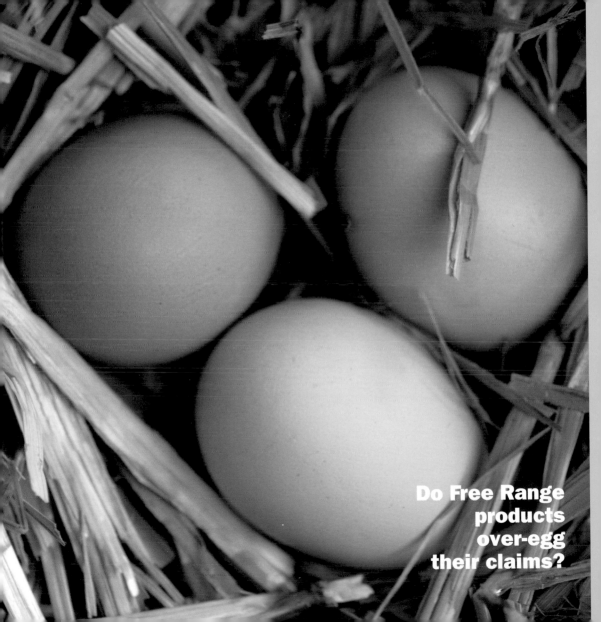

Do Free Range
products
over-egg
their claims?

short-term memory, according to a study in the *European Journal of Clinical Nutrition*. Not what you need just before your important morning meeting with the boss.

The truth about...
COLOURED SWEETS

Skittles say they allow you to "taste the rainbow?" We're not sure what rainbows are made of (light?), but we doubt it's the unsettling mash-up of sugar, glucose syrup, and Carnauba Wax (the same wax used for car and shoe polish) used to construct these neon orbs. All in all, each little packet contains more sugar than a Mars bar and nearly every gram of fat in Skittles is saturated.

To achieve that colour spectrum, manufacturers brings in a whole new list of additives. So, when you taste those different flavours what you're really tasting is the laboratory constructed amalgam of artificial colours, many of which have been linked to behavioural and attention deficit problems in children. A few years ago *The Lancet* published a study linking these artificial additives to hyperactivity and behavioural problems in children. This prompted the Food Standards Agency to call for an EU-wide labelling system and for the dyes to be phased out. Nevertheless many food manufacturers continue to use them. Consumers are advised to check ingredients for prime offenders such as tartrazine (E102), quinoline yellow (E104).

The truth about...
ENERGY DRINKS

These beverages boast exotic-sounding supplements and make superhuman claims: long-lasting energy! Boosted concentration! Increased athletic performance! But do they really rev up your body and sharpen your mind?

The jolt you'll feel from downing one of these energy elixirs comes from a combination of sky-high caffeine levels and staggering sugar content. Added extras, like ginseng, guarana, and taurine, make minimal difference. Ginseng might boost your brainpower (Australia's Swinburne University of Technology found people who had the extract before taking a cognitive test scored better than when they skipped the supplement) but it won't boost energy levels. Guarana's benefit comes from its caffeine content—a guarana seed contains 4 to 5 percent caffeine (about twice as much as a coffee bean).

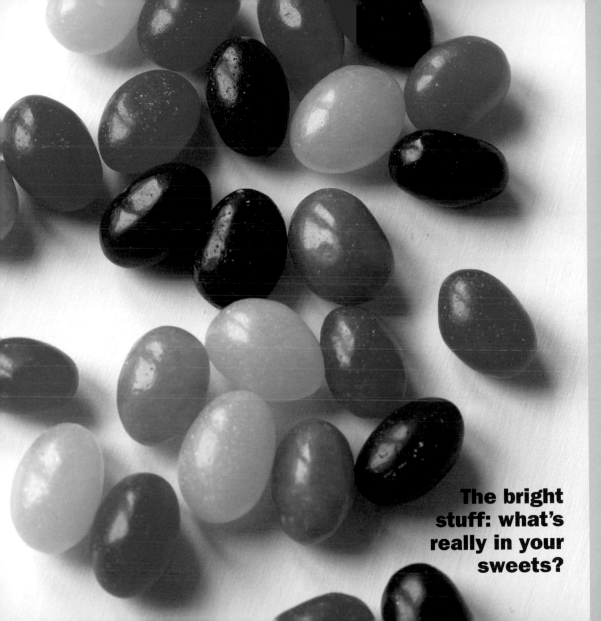

The bright stuff: what's really in your sweets?

And taurine (an additive in Red Bull) actually might make you feel sluggish, not hyperactive, according to researchers at Weill Cornell Medical College. As for that "long-lasting" energy? If your drink is packed with sugar (and most of them are), you're bound for a crash. Seems counterproductive, doesn't it?

The truth about...
SALAMI
Salami, the mystery meat: Is it cow? Is it pig? Well, if you're talking fast food Genoa salami, then it's often both. Most mass-produced salami is made from slaughterhouse leftovers that are gathered using a technique called "advanced meat recovery," which sounds like a rehab centre for vegans, but is actually a mechanical process that strips the last of the remaining bits of muscle off the bone so nothing is wasted. It's then processed using lactic acid, the waste product produced by bacteria in the meat. It both gives the salami its tangy flavour and cures it as well, making it an inhospitable place for any other bacteria to grow. Add in a bunch of salt and spices and you've got salami. Now that you know

what's in there, you might want to opt for the chicken sandwich next time, or even go veggie.

The truth about...
CRISPS
Britain has more flavours of crisp than anywhere else in the world. Fat and calories vary from brand to brand, but once you open a bag, you tend to keep munching until there is nothing left. So why are crisps so addictive?

Well, before the fats and carbs reach your stomach, your taste buds will enjoy the seasoning blend, which may include sugar, "artificial flavouring," and worrisome compound called monosodium glutamate. Monosodium glutamate, or MSG, is the flavour enhancer largely responsible for the addictive quality of many brands of crisp. The drawback is that it interferes with the production of an appetite-regulating hormone called leptin. That's why a study of published in the journal *Obesity* found a strong correlation between MSG consumption and body fat. What's worse; every year medical complaints come from people who react violently to MSG, suffering symptoms such as nausea, headaches, numbness and chest pains.

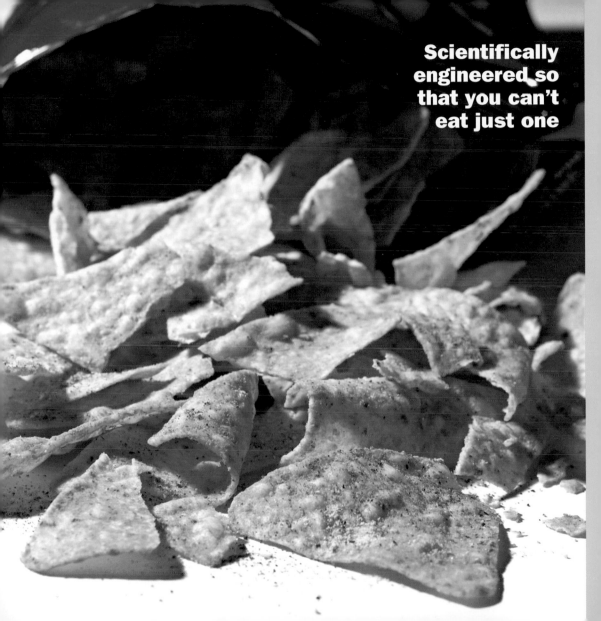

Scientifically engineered so that you can't eat just one

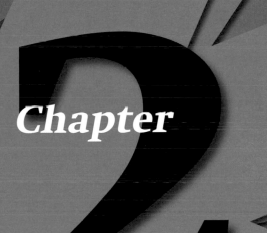

Chapter 2

FOODS THAT CURE

You might think,

after skimming a few chapters in this book, that we'd like nothing more than to stop you eating food altogether. And you might think, after surveying the UK's current dietary landscape, that that's not such a bad idea.

After all, it's hard to escape the reality of Britain's growing obesity problem—especially after a day on the beach, when you watch a crowd of environmentally conscious children trying to save a beached whale, only to discover it's just a pale, middle-aged guy in Speedos who's had one too many mojitos. Or after an evening on the sofa watching the latest debate over the NHS, when you realise that if our food supply weren't so tainted by lard-laden junk, we wouldn't be lumbered with a bill of over £4 billion a year just to treat the UK's weight problem. You might think the solution is to put the whole country on a diet and make everybody stop eating so many meals and so many snacks.

But eating too much food isn't the problem. The problem is that we're eating too many things that aren't actually food—the additives, the preservatives, the chemically enhanced foodlike substances. And even when we do eat real food, those meals and snacks are often served in such calorie-loaded portions that even our old-fashioned grandmothers who always told us to "eat up" would step back, aghast, and shout, "Take that out of your mouth!"

But in reality, food—*real* food—is a good thing. Real food, the kind that comes from the earth rather than a science lab, is about more than just calories and carbs, salts and sugars. Real food can have almost magical properties—amazing abilities to prevent or even heal many of our physical and emotional woes.

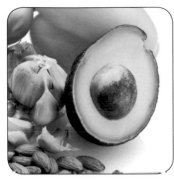 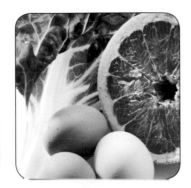 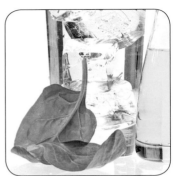

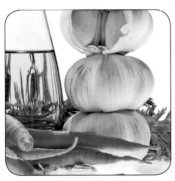 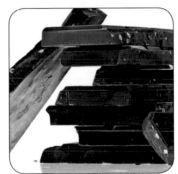 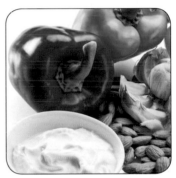

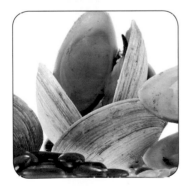 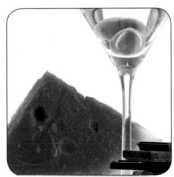 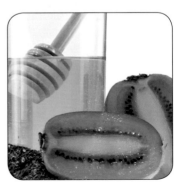

Our bodies are designed to function at their optimum levels and to look and feel lean, strong, and vibrant when they're fed the vitamins, minerals, healthy fats, and micronutrients found in real food.

Imagine, if you will, a happier more positive world with less stress and less frustration. It would look a lot like today's world, except for two things: (1) Jack Dee would be out of a job, and (2) the rest of us would be dining on salmon, washing it down with a glass of wine, and snacking on dark chocolate for dessert. Those three things have been shown in studies to brighten our moods and beat back the fatigue and depression so many of us labour under.

But chances are irritable comedians will have plenty to bemoan in coming years, as long as they and the rest of us keep chowing down on foods that are high in carbs, high in fat, and high in preservatives. And we will continue to battle weight issues as well because all of those bad-for-you foodstuffs set us up for even more hunger and even more weight gain.

But eating lots and lots of healthy foods can help you lose weight—in fact, it's a much better way to keep off extra pounds than not eating anything at all.

That's because our bodies are designed not only to enjoy real food and to thrive on the nutrients within, but also to burn off the calories in real food and drink. Indeed, eating smart throughout the day revs up your body's metabolism—the internal fat furnace that turns calories into energy—and gives you all-day get-up-and-go energy. Stop feeding yourself good food and your body goes into starvation mode, saving calories like a miser—except instead of storing them under a mattress, you'll be storing them in your belly, your chin(s), and other unsightly hiding places.

So, we're outlining the best foods for whatever ails you and explaining exactly how these mealtime miracle workers will improve your looks, your life, and even your attitude. This is your ultimate cure-all nutritional prescription.

When You're Stressed

Eat This
FRIED EGGS

Go ahead, crack under pressure: eating fried eggs may help reduce high blood pressure. In a test-tube study, scientists in Canada discovered that the breakfast standby produced the highest levels of ACE inhibitory peptides. These amino acids dilate blood vessels, allowing your blood to flow more easily.

WINE

It's true: A glass of wine really does take the edge off. But you may want to stop there. Researchers from the University of Toronto discovered that one alcoholic drink caused people's blood vessels to relax, but two drinks began to reverse the benefits. That's because when your blood alcohol content reaches a certain level, your central nervous system releases noradrenaline— the same hormone released when you're in high stress.

GUM

When you find yourself feeling overwhelmed at work, reach for the Wrigley's: chewing gum can tame your tension, according to Australian researchers. People who chewed gum while taking multitasking tests reported a 17 percent drop in stress. This might have something to do with the fact that we associate chewing with positive social interactions, such as mealtimes.

Not That!
COFFEE

A cup of joe can cut through your morning mental fog, but too much coffee could worsen your work anxiety, found research from the University of Oklahoma. The scientists found that when people downed the caffeine equivalent of three cups of java, their symptoms of psychological stress increased. Caffeine triggers a rise in your blood level of cortisol, the hormone released when you feel threatened.

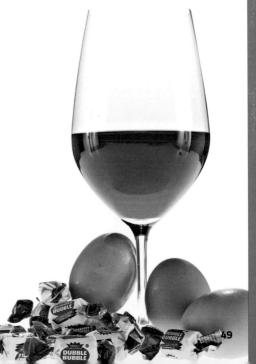

When You're Feeling Down

⬏ Eat This
SALMON

Omega-3s may calm your neurotic side, according to a study in the journal *Psychosomatic Medicine*. Researchers found that adults with the lowest blood levels of eicosapentaenoic acid (EPA) and docosahexaenoic acid (DHA) were more likely to have neuroses, which are symptoms for depression. EPA and DHA are key brain components, and higher levels of each can bolster the potent mood enhancers serotonin and dopamine. Salmon is loaded with EPA and DHA, as are walnuts, flaxseeds, and cauliflower.

⬏ GARLIC

Throw a few extra cloves into your next stir-fry or pasta sauce: research has found that enzymes in garlic can help increase the release of serotonin, a neurochemical that makes you feel relaxed. Plus, garlic may have the added benefit of improving memory. Pakistani researchers found that rats fed a puree of garlic and water performed better on a memory test than rats that weren't fed the mixture.

⬏ DARK CHOCOLATE

Research shows that dark chocolate can improve heart health, lower blood pressure and reduce LDL cholesterol. It also boosts serotonin and endorphin levels, which are associated with improved mood and greater concentration. Look for chocolate that is 60 percent cocoa or higher.

⬏ Not That!
WHITE CHOCOLATE

Now technically, white chocolate isn't chocolate, since it contains no cocoa solids. Instead, it's made mostly with fats and sugar, lacking the nutritional vigour of the real stuff. That means it also lacks the ability to stimulate the euphoria-inducing chemicals that real chocolate does—especially serotonin.

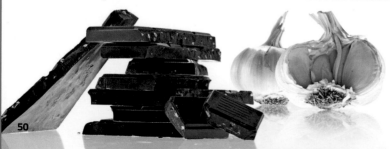

When You Want to Boost Your Metabolism

⮨ Eat This

CHILLI PEPPERS

It turns out that capsaicin, the compound that gives chillis their mouth-searing quality, is also what causes it to fire up your metabolism. Eating about 1 tablespoon of chopped red or green chillis boosts the amount of heat your body produces and activates your sympathetic nervous system (responsible for our fight-or-flight response), found a study in the *Journal of Nutritional Science and Vitaminology.* The result? A metabolism spike of up to 23 percent.

⮨ CAFFEINATED COFFEE

A study published in the journal *Physiology and Behavior* found that the average metabolic rate of people who drank caffeinated coffee increased 16 percent over those who drank decaf. This is because caffeine increases your heart rate and breathing, which stimulates your central nervous system.

⮨ YOGURT

The probiotics in yogurt may speed weight loss. British scientists found that these active organisms boosted the breakdown of fat molecules in mice, which prevented the rodents from gaining weight. Try the Horizon brand of yogurt— it contains the probiotic *L. casei,* the same organism used in the study.

⮨ Not That!

NOTHING

That's right: There's no better way to grind your metabolism to a halt than skipping a meal. When your body goes without food, it switches into survival mode, storing calories rather than burning them. Breakfast is most important, because your body is still in shutdown mode and your metabolism needs a strong protein-and fibre-based jump start.

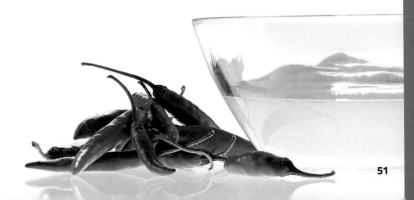

When You Need More Energy

CLAMS

Clams stock your body with magnesium, which is important in metabolism, nerve function, and muscle function. When magnesium levels are low, your body produces more lactic acid—the same fatigue-inducing substance that you feel at the end of a long workout.

GRILLED CHICKEN BREAST

The protein in lean meat like chicken, fish, or pork loin won't just squash your hunger and boost your metabolism, it's also a top source of energy. University of Illinois researchers found people who ate more protein had higher energy levels and didn't feel as tired as those who ate a higher proportion of carbs in their diet.

KIDNEY BEANS

These legumes are a great source of thiamin and riboflavin. Both vitamins help your body use energy efficiently, so you won't be nodding off mid PowerPoint.

BARLEY

Swedish researchers found that if you eat barley for breakfast, the fibrous grain cuts blood sugar response by 44 percent at lunch and 14 percent at dinner. And the less your sugar spikes, the more stable your energy levels will be.

Not That! BAGELS

Researchers from the Massachusetts Institute of Technology analysed blood samples from people who had eaten either a high-protein or a high-carb breakfast. Two hours after eating, the carb eaters had tryptophan levels 14 percent higher than before, whereas protein eaters decreased their tryptophan levels by 28 percent. The higher your tryptophan level, the more likely you are to feel tired and sluggish. So less of the toast and muffins, and more of the eggs and bacon.

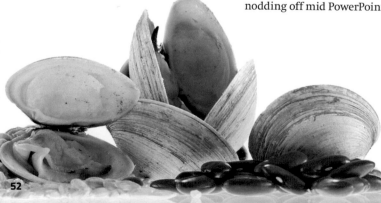

When You're Sick

Eat This
KIWI

The vitamin C in kiwi won't prevent the onslaught of a cold, but it might decrease the duration of your symptoms. One kiwi fruit provides 117 percent of your recommended daily amount of vitamin C.

HONEY

Pennsylvania State University scientists have discovered that honey can act as a powerful cough suppressant—so next time you're hacking up a lung, head for the kitchen. When parents of 105 sick children doled out honey or dextromethorphan (the active ingredient in most cough medicines), the honey was better at lessening cough frequency and severity. Try a drizzle in a cup of tea.

ROOIBOS TEA

Animal research suggests that this South African tea may provide potent immunity-boosting benefits. Large human studies have yet to be conducted, though.

OLIVES

Foods rich in healthy fats help reduce inflammation, a catalyst for migraines. One study found the anti-inflammatory compounds in olive oil can suppress the enzymes involved in inflammation in the same manner as ibuprofen. Avocados and almonds are also high in monoun-saturated fats.

Not That!
CAFFEINATED BEVERAGES AND ENERGY DRINKS

Caffeine can mess with your sleep schedule, and lack of sleep opens the door to colds, upper respiratory infections, and other ills. What's more, caffeine is dehydrating, and hydration is vital during illness: not only do fluids transport nutrients to the illness site but they also help dispose of toxins.

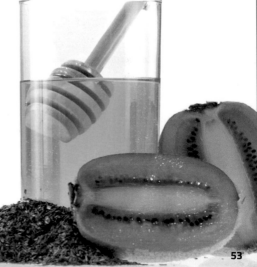

When You Want to Get in the Mood

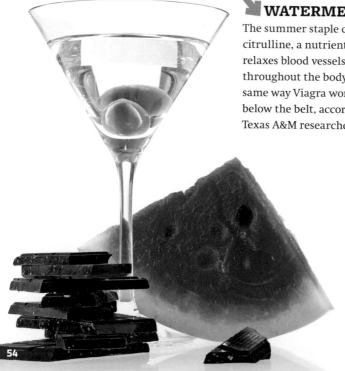

Eat This
DARK CHOCOLATE

Chocolate is packed with the compounds anandamide and phenylethylamine, which cause the body to release the same feel-good endorphins triggered by sex and physical exertion. Cocoa also contains methylxanthines, which make skin more sensitive to touch.

WATERMELON

The summer staple contains citrulline, a nutrient that relaxes blood vessels throughout the body in the same way Viagra works below the belt, according to Texas A&M researchers.

ALCOHOL

Booze acts as a depressant in the brain's cerebral cortex, lowering inhibitions that could otherwise restrain arousal. However, when men consumed too much, their erections weren't as strong as when they had limited themselves to just one or two drinks.

Not That!
OYSTERS

OK, they won't exactly inhibit your bedroom behaviour, but these legendary "aphrodisiacs" have never been proven to actually boost libido. While zinc, abundant in oysters of all shapes and sizes, is linked to male fertility, the connections to actual arousal have never been borne out in clinical research.

When You Work Out

⬊ Eat This
SPINACH

In a test-tube study, Rutgers researchers discovered that treating human muscle cells with a compound found in spinach increased protein synthesis by 20 percent. The compound allows muscle tissue to repair itself faster, the researchers say.

⬊ GREEN TEA

Brazilian scientists found that participants who consumed three cups of the beverage every day for a week had fewer markers of the cell damage caused by resistance to exercise. That means that green tea can help you recover faster after an intense workout.

⬊ CHOCOLATE MILK SHAKE

Nothing like a little dessert after a long workout. British researchers found chocolate milk does a better job than sports drinks when it comes to replenishing the body after a workout. Why? Because it has higher levels of electrolytes and a higher fat content. Scientists at James Madison University found that the balance of fat, protein, and carbs in chocolate milk makes it nearly one-third more effective at replenishing muscles than other recovery beverages. And, of course, don't forget H_2O: even as little as a 1 percent decrease in your body water can impair your performance when exercising.

⬊ FISH OIL

Australian researchers found that cyclists who took fish oil for eight weeks had lower heart rates and consumed less oxygen during intense cycling than a control group.

⬊ Not That!
RED BULL

Caffeine may be a proven training aid, but drinking a Red Bull won't provide enough stimulation to affect your workouts, according to Canadian studies. A group of fit adults who drank up to two cans of the drink an hour before a sprint didn't experience a performance boost. The beverage doesn't provide enough of a jolt.

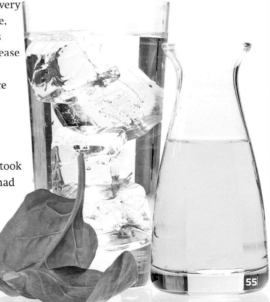

When You Need a Brain Boost...

...For Focus

⬇ Eat This
SARDINES

According to research in the *Nutrition Journal,* fish oil increases your ability to concentrate. Credit EPA and DHA—fatty acids that bolster communication among brain cells and help regulate neurotransmitters responsible for mental focus. Can't stomach sardines at your desk? Try a handful of omega-3 rich walnuts instead.

⬇ Not That!
SWEETS

Sugary foods provoke sudden surges of glucose that result big in highs and lows in your energy levels. Unfortunately, the lows outlast the highs, as do the possible headaches and lack of concentration.

...For Improved Memory

⬇ Eat This
GARLIC

Researchers in Pakistan found that rats fed on a puree of garlic and water performed better on memory tests than rats that weren't fed the mixture. That's because garlic increases the brain's levels of serotonin, which has been shown to enhance memory function.

⬇ BANANAS

The antioxidants in bananas, apples and oranges may help protect you from Alzheimer's, report Korean scientists. In a test-tube study, the researchers found that plant chemicals known as polyphenols could help to shield brain cells from oxidative stress—a key cause of the disease.

⬎ Not That!
SOFT DRINKS

Spikes in blood sugar can wreck short-term memory, according to a study in the *European Journal of Clinical Nutrition*. Scientists tested adults who had just downed a sugary drink, those with the highest blood glucose levels had the worst recall. Fizzy drinks are an obvious offender, but many "juice" drinks are loaded down with a rush of added sugars and glucose-fructose syrup.

⬎ ENERGY DRINKS AND COFFEE

Like a politician whose smile is just a little too eager, caffeine has a dark side, too. Too much of it can make you jittery, anxious, and unsure of yourself. It can also derail your sleep schedule, which means that extra cup of coffee today can blunt your cognitive powers tomorrow.

...For Lasting Brainpower

⬎ Eat This
STEAK

Vitamin B12, an essential nutrient found in meat, milk, and fish, may protect you against brain degeneration as you age, say British scientists. The researchers found that older people with the highest blood levels of the vitamin were six times less likely to have brain shrinkage than those with the lowest levels.

⬎ CARROTS

Researchers from Harvard found that men who consumed higher levels of beta-carotene over 18 years had significantly delayed cognitive ageing. Carrots are a tremendous source of the antioxidant, as are other orange foods such as peppers, butternut squash and pumpkins.

...For Sharper Senses

⬎ Eat This
GROUND FLAXSEED

Flax is the best source of alpha-linolenic acid (ALA)—a healthy fat that improves the workings of the cerebral cortex, the area of the brain that processes sensory information, including that of pleasure. To meet your quota, just sprinkle 1 tablespoon of flaxseed on salads or cereal once a day, or mix it into a smoothie or shake.

⬎ Not That!
ALCOHOL

This one's obvious, but worth stressing anyway. While a drink or two can increase arousal signals, more than a few drinks will actually depress your nervous system. This will dull sensations and make you tired, not sharp—in your brain and throughout the rest of your body.

10 Foods You Should Eat Every Day

We talk a lot about the foods you can't eat in this book—foods so infused with calories, fat and salt they should come with warnings like the ones on cigarette packets. With many of us eating on the go, it often seems our choice is limited to the lesser of two fast-food evils, and all the textbook nutritious stuff doesn't even get a look in. However, the 10 foods highlighted below are all easy to incorporate into your diet—and are capable not just of helping to boost your metabolism and melt fat, but also of fighting disease, lowering cholesterol, stabilising blood sugar, and helping you to live a longer life. And did we mention that they're delicious? Make it your goal to work these superfoods into your day.

1. EGGS

When it comes to breakfast, you can't beat eggs. (That was too easy, wasn't it?) Seriously though, at a cost of only 72 calories, each large egg holds 6.3 grams of high-quality protein, along with a powerhouse punch of vital nutrients. A study published in the *International Journal of Obesity* found that people who replaced carbs with eggs for breakfast lost as much as 65 percent more weight. Research conducted in Michigan showed that regular egg eaters enjoyed more vitamins and minerals in their diets than those who ate few or no eggs. By examining surveys from more than 27,000 people, the researchers found that egg eaters were about half as likely to be deficient in vitamin B12, 24 percent less likely to be deficient in vitamin A, and 36 percent less likely to be deficient in vitamin E. And here's something more surprising: those who ate at least four eggs a week had noticeably lower cholesterol levels than those who ate fewer than one. Turns out the dietary cholesterol in the yolk has little impact on your levels of blood cholesterol.
Substitutes None

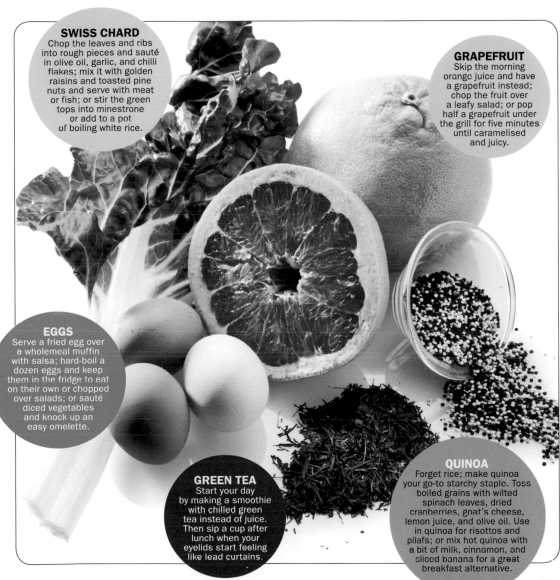

SWISS CHARD
Chop the leaves and ribs into rough pieces and sauté in olive oil, garlic, and chilli flakes; mix it with golden raisins and toasted pine nuts and serve with meat or fish; or stir the green tops into minestrone or add to a pot of boiling white rice.

GRAPEFRUIT
Skip the morning orange juice and have a grapefruit instead; chop the fruit over a leafy salad; or pop half a grapefruit under the grill for five minutes until caramelised and juicy.

EGGS
Serve a fried egg over a wholemeal muffin with salsa; hard-boil a dozen eggs and keep them in the fridge to eat on their own or chopped over salads; or sauté diced vegetables and knock up an easy omelette.

GREEN TEA
Start your day by making a smoothie with chilled green tea instead of juice. Then sip a cup after lunch when your eyelids start feeling like lead curtains.

QUINOA
Forget rice; make quinoa your go-to starchy staple. Toss boiled grains with wilted spinach leaves, dried cranberries, goat's cheese, lemon juice, and olive oil. Use in quinoa for risottos and pilafs; or mix hot quinoa with a bit of milk, cinnamon, and sliced banana for a great breakfast alternative.

59

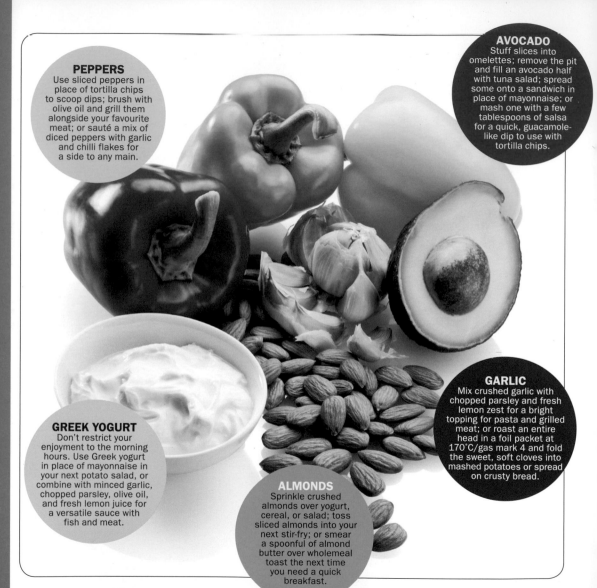

PEPPERS
Use sliced peppers in place of tortilla chips to scoop dips; brush with olive oil and grill them alongside your favourite meat; or sauté a mix of diced peppers with garlic and chilli flakes for a side to any main.

AVOCADO
Stuff slices into omelettes; remove the pit and fill an avocado half with tuna salad; spread some onto a sandwich in place of mayonnaise; or mash one with a few tablespoons of salsa for a quick, guacamole-like dip to use with tortilla chips.

GARLIC
Mix crushed garlic with chopped parsley and fresh lemon zest for a bright topping for pasta and grilled meat; or roast an entire head in a foil packet at 170°C/gas mark 4 and fold the sweet, soft cloves into mashed potatoes or spread on crusty bread.

GREEK YOGURT
Don't restrict your enjoyment to the morning hours. Use Greek yogurt in place of mayonnaise in your next potato salad, or combine with minced garlic, chopped parsley, olive oil, and fresh lemon juice for a versatile sauce with fish and meat.

ALMONDS
Sprinkle crushed almonds over yogurt, cereal, or salad; toss sliced almonds into your next stir-fry; or smear a spoonful of almond butter over wholemeal toast the next time you need a quick breakfast.

2. GREEN TEA

Literally thousands of studies have been carried out to document the health benefits of catechins, the group of antioxidants concentrated in the leaves of tea plants. Among the most startling studies was one published by the American Medical Association in 2006. The study followed more than 40,000 Japanese adults for a decade, and at the 7-year follow-up, those who had been drinking five or more cups of tea per day were 26 percent less likely to die of any cause compared with those who averaged less than a cup. Looking for more immediate results? Another Japanese study broke participants into two groups, only one of which was put on a catechin-rich green-tea diet. At the end of 12 weeks, the green-tea group had achieved significantly smaller body weights and waistlines than those in the control group. Why? Because researchers believe that catechins are effective at boosting metabolism.

Substitutes Yerba mate, white tea, oolong tea, rooibos (red) tea

3. GARLIC

Allicin, an antibacterial and antifungal compound, is the steam engine pushing forward garlic's health benefits. The chemical is produced by the garlic plant as a defence against pests, but inside your body it fights cancer, strengthens your cardiovascular system, decreases fat storage, and fights acne. To activate it crush the garlic as finely as possible. Peel the cloves, then use the side of a heavy chef's knife to squash it before carefully crushing or chopping. Then be sure not to overcook it, as too much heat will render the compound completely useless (and your food with a bitter aftertaste).

Substitutes Onions, chives, leeks

4. GRAPEFRUIT

Just call it the better-body fruit. In a study of 100 obese people at the Scripps Clinic in California, those who ate half a grapefruit with each meal lost an average of 3.6 pounds (1.6 kilos) over the course of 12 weeks. Many lost more than 10 pounds. The study's control group, in contrast, lost a paltry ½ pound. But here's something better: those who ate the grapefruit also exhibited a decrease in insulin levels, indicating that their bodies had improved upon the ability to metabolise sugar. If you can't stomach a grapefruit a day, try to find as many ways possible to sneak grapefruit into your diet. Even a moderate increase in grapefruit intake should yield results, not to mention earning you a massive dose of lycopene—the cancer-preventing antioxidant found most commonly in tomatoes.

Substitutes Oranges, watermelon, tomatoes

5. GREEK YOGURT

Regular yogurt is more of a dessert than a meal. If you want substance, go Greek. What sets the two apart? Greek yogurt is separated from the watery whey that sits on top of regular yogurt, and the process removes excessive sugars such as lactose and increases the concentration of protein by as much as three times. That means it fills your belly more like a meal than a snack. Plus half a big pot has almost a quarter of your day's calcium, and studies show calcium-rich diets can help you to lose body fat. In one of these studies, participants on a high-calcium dairy diet were able to lose 70 percent more body weight than those on a calorie-restricted diet alone. If only everything you ate could make a similar claim.

Substitutes Kefir and yogurt with "live and active cultures" printed on the product label

6. AVOCADO

Here's what often gets lost in our fat phobia: Some of those fats are actually good for you. More than half the calories in each creamy green fruit comes from one of the world's healthiest fats, monounsaturates. These fats differ from saturated fats in that they have one double-bonded carbon atom, but that small difference at the molecular level amounts to a dramatic improvement to your health. Numerous studies have shown that monounsaturated fats both improve your cholesterol profile and decrease the amount of triglycerides (more bad fats) floating around in your blood. That can lower your risk of stroke and heart disease. Worried about weight gain? Don't be. There's no causal link between monounsaturated fats and body fat.

Substitutes Olive, canola and peanut oils, peanut butter, tahini

7. QUINOA

Although not yet common in British kitchens, quinoa (pronounced keen-wa) boasts more nutrients than any other grain. It has more fibre and nearly twice as much protein as brown rice, and the proteins it has consist of a near-perfect blend of amino acids, so that your body can easily break them down and turn them into muscle. And get this: All that protein and fibre— in conjunction with a handful of healthy fats and a comparatively small dose of carbohydrates—help ensure a low impact on your blood sugar. That's great news for prediabetics and anyone watching their weight. So what's the trade-off? There is none. Quinoa's soft and nutty taste is easy to handle even for picky eaters, and it cooks just like rice, ready in about 15 minutes.

Substitutes Oats, amaranth, millet, pearl barley, bulgur wheat

8. PEPPERS

All peppers are loaded with antioxidants, but none so much as the brightly coloured reds, yellows, and oranges. These colours result from carotenoids concentrated in the flesh of the pepper, the same carotenoids that give tomatoes, carrots, and grapefruits their healthy hues. The range of benefits provided by these pigments include improved cell communication, better immune system function, protection against sun damage, and a diminished risk for several types of cancer. And if you can take the heat, try cooking with chilli peppers, too. They're still loaded with carotenoids and vitamin C but have the added benefit of capsaicins, temperature-raising phytochemicals that fight headache and arthritis pain as well as boost metabolism.
Substitutes Carrots, sweet potatoes, watermelon

9. ALMONDS

Thirty grams of almonds a day, about 23 nuts, provides 9 grams of heart-healthy oleic acid, which is more than peanuts, walnuts, or cashews. This monounsaturated fat is known to be responsible for many health benefits, the most recently discovered of which is improved memory. Rats in California were better able to navigate a maze the second time around if they'd been fed oleic acid, and there's no reason to assume that the same treatment won't help you navigate your day-to-day life. If nothing else, snacking on them will take your mind off your hunger. Nearly a quarter of an almond's calories come from fibre and protein. Researchers at Purdue University found this is made a group who ate the nuts feel full for an hour and a half longer than a group who at rice cakes.
Substitutes Walnuts, pecans, peanuts, sesame seeds, flaxseeds

10. SWISS CHARD

Most fruits and vegetables are role players, supplying us with a monster dose of a single nutrient. But Swiss chard is nature's multivitamin, delivering substantial amounts of 16 vitamins and vital nutrients, and it does so at a rock-bottom caloric cost. For a mere 35 calories' worth of cooked chard, you get more than 716 percent of your recommended daily intake of bone-strengthening vitamin K, 214 percent of your day's vitamin A (to defend against cancer and bolster vision), and 17 percent of hard-to-get vitamin E (which can help sharpen mental acuity). Plus, emerging research suggests that Swiss chard's combination of fibre and phytonutrients and may provide an effective defence against colon cancer.
Substitutes Spinach, mustard greens, watercress, arugula, romaine lettuce

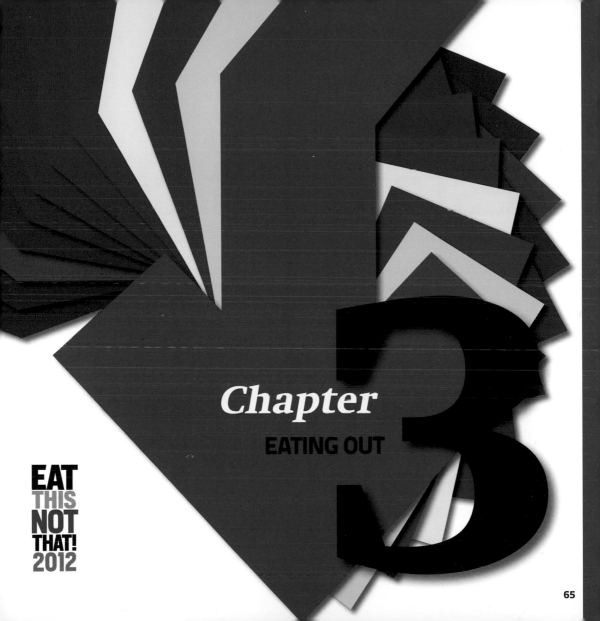

Chapter

EATING OUT

EAT
THIS
NOT
THAT!
2012

Restaurant chefs

make cookery look so romantic on television. You could go one-on-one with Gordon Ramsay on *Hell's Kitchen,* find a recipe to melt John Torode and Gregg Wallace's heart's on *MasterChef,* travel the world feasting on exotic foods like Rick Stein does on *Taste The Blues* or watch Jamie Oliver take on the establishment from a kitchen. Foodie television makes it seem as though anyone with a ladle and a spatula is a swashbuckling culinary cavalier.

The reality is very different. The vast majority of professional cooks in the United Kingdom don't work under wild-eyed slave drivers, whipping up ingenious new recipes out of sheep heart, bull testicles, and bok choy and wowing their customers with stunning new taste sensations. The average cook works in your local Bella Italia, or Nando's, or Wetherspoons, and the *last* thing their boss or their customers want is for them to get *creative*. Indeed, the cooks at the Little Chef in Milton Keynes are cooking the exact same ingredients in the exact same way as their compatriots in Middlewich. Uniformity, not creativity, is the key to modern restaurant success.

So when it comes to knowing exactly what's in your restaurant meal—and how many calories you're consuming when you eat it—you'd think getting the facts would be pretty easy. After all, they're using the same stuff in every Little Chef Olympic Breakfast from Land's End to John O'Groats.

Yet many restaurant chains refuse to tell their customers what it is, exactly, that they're putting into their bodies, claiming that it's just too hard to work out. But one thing we've learned is this: nobody hesitates to tell you *good* news. During our research process for this, the first UK edition of *Eat This, Not That!*, we looked extensively for nutritional values, and often found claims of healthy food, but then, on closer investigation, found no dietary information to back it up.

Some seem to be making an effort. Growing chain Giraffe, for instance, told us their information would be published "soon", as did Little Chef, although they couldn't give us an exact date. We're hoping it will be ready for the next edition of this book. Others were completely dismissive. Wagamama, for instance, state on their website, "We currently do not have any plans to release nutritional information on our dishes, but remain committed to providing fresh and nutritious food at all times to our customers." Well that answers that. Don't ask, don't tell.

And although us Brits may take some comfort in our slightly lower obesity levels when compared to the US (1 in 4 here, as opposed to 1 in 3 in over there) how long can it stay that way when we actually have less nutritional information than they do? Some of the franchise restaurants that have made it across the pond (TGI Friday's, Hard Rock Cafe, Papa John's) seem to have lost their nutritional information on the voyage. So even if our American cousins are eating too much, at least they know what's on their plates. Why shouldn't we?

Trusting a multinational corporation to put things into your body—and then not being able to find out exactly what those things are—sounds like a foolhardy enterprise (and maybe the plot to a Stephen King novel). So for this chapter, *Eat This, Not That!* has dug deep and revealed the secrets that many big chains don't want you to know. Whether you're in the mood for pizza, pasta, pies or something smothered in peri peri everything you need to know is on these pages...

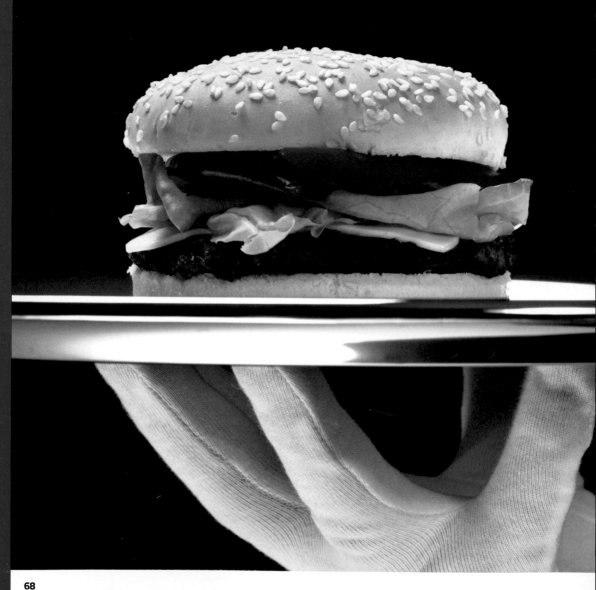

In every sandwich shop and burger joint there are healthy options (and not so healthy ones). This guide will help you to navigate the nutritional minefield

Fast
Food

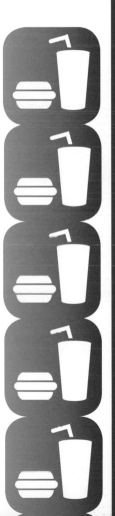

Burger King

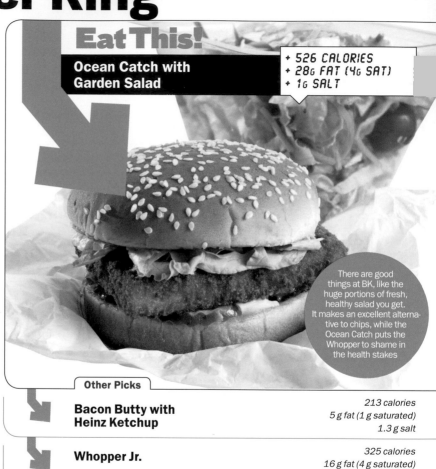

The King holds the crown for being one of the trickier places to find something healthy on the menu, but seek and ye shall find. Surprisingly good for you are the chicken nuggets, which make a better side dish than either fries or onion rings. Avoid the Smoked Bacon and Cheddar Double Angus at all costs. 966 calories and 23 grams of saturated fat in one burger? It's just unnecessary...

SURVIVAL STRATEGY

For breakfast, pick the Bacon Butty with either ketchup or HP. For lunch, match the Hamburger with six chicken nuggets and water and you'll do both meals for less than 800 calories in total.

Eat This!

Ocean Catch with Garden Salad

+ 526 CALORIES
+ 28G FAT (4G SAT)
+ 1G SALT

There are good things at BK, like the huge portions of fresh, healthy salad you get. It makes an excellent alternative to chips, while the Ocean Catch puts the Whopper to shame in the health stakes

Other Picks

Bacon Butty with Heinz Ketchup

213 calories
5 g fat (1 g saturated)
1.3 g salt

Whopper Jr.

325 calories
16 g fat (4 g saturated)
1.45 g salt

Chicken Nuggets x 6

258 calories
13 g fat (3.7 g saturated)
1.45 g salt

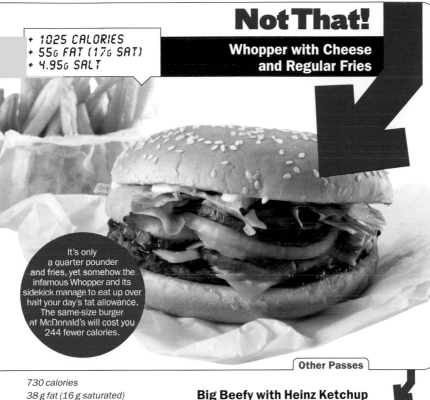

+ 1025 CALORIES
+ 55G FAT (17G SAT)
+ 4.95G SALT

Not That!

Whopper with Cheese and Regular Fries

It's only a quarter pounder and fries, yet somehow the infamous Whopper and its sidekick manage to eat up over half your day's fat allowance. The same-size burger at McDonald's will cost you 244 fewer calories.

Other Passes

730 calories
38 g fat (16 g saturated)
3.67 g salt

Big Beefy with Heinz Ketchup

966 calories
58 g fat (23 g saturated)
2.65 g salt

Smoked Bacon & Cheddar Double Angus

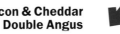

398 calories
20 g fat (3 g saturated,)
0.3 g salt

Onion Rings
(regular)

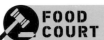

FOOD COURT

THE CRIME
Double Whopper with Cheese
(976 calories)

THE PUNISHMENT
Pedal vigorously (at about 15mph) on an exercise bike for an hour

 LITTLE TRICK

Have a burger without mayo and you'll save over 100 calories and 10 grams of fat.

 GUILTY PLEASURE

Sweet Chilli Chicken Wrap
296 calories
6 g fat
(2 g saturated)

This beats even chicken nuggets with its extremely low fat content. It also has around 50 fewer calories than its innocent sounding cousin the Caesar Chicken Wrap. All this plus 23 grams of muscle-building protein. Maximise your pleasure.

Caffè Nero

The high-street coffee chain gets bonus points in the health stakes for helpfully flagging up which of its sandwiches are low in calories. Virtually all of them are under 500 calories and as we went to press their range had two under 300 calories, which is more than enough reason to drop in for your lunch. As ever with coffee shops avoid the creamy, flavoured drinks at all costs. Don't like the taste of coffee? Have a tea.

SURVIVAL STRATEGY

Make this your coffee shop—it has some of the lowest calorie hot drinks around thanks to its using semi-skimmed milk.

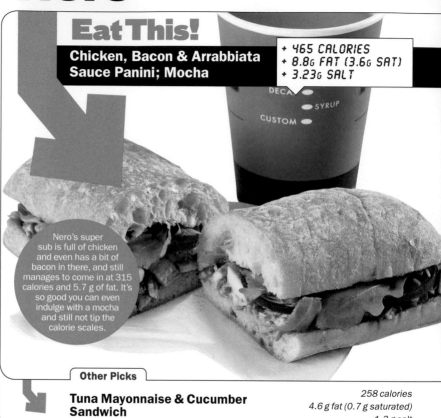

Eat This!

Chicken, Bacon & Arrabbiata Sauce Panini; Mocha

+ 465 CALORIES
+ 8.8G FAT (3.6G SAT)
+ 3.23G SALT

Nero's super sub is full of chicken and even has a bit of bacon in there, and still manages to come in at 315 calories and 5.7 g of fat. It's so good you can even indulge with a mocha and still not tip the calorie scales.

Other Picks

Tuna Mayonnaise & Cucumber Sandwich
258 calories
4.6 g fat (0.7 g saturated)
1.3 g salt

Chicken Salad Sandwich
272 calories
4.2 g fat (0.6 g saturated)
1 g salt

Latte, regular
69 calories
2.6 g fat (1.7 g saturated)
7.1 g sugar

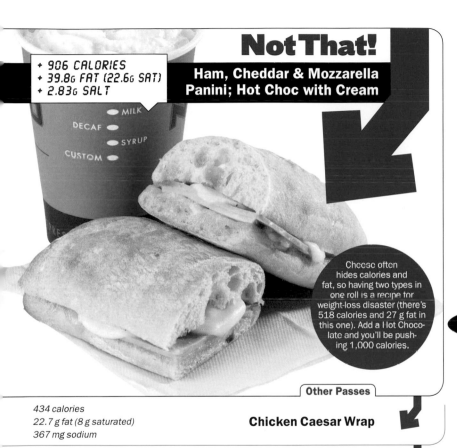

Not That!

Ham, Cheddar & Mozzarella Panini; Hot Choc with Cream

- 906 CALORIES
- 39.8G FAT (22.6G SAT)
- 2.83G SALT

MILK
DECAF
SYRUP
CUSTOM

Cheese often hides calories and fat, so having two types in one roll is a recipe for weight-loss disaster (there's 518 calories and 27 g fat in this one). Add a Hot Chocolate and you'll be pushing 1,000 calories.

Other Passes

434 calories 22.7 g fat (8 g saturated) 367 mg sodium	**Chicken Caesar Wrap**
424 calories 21.8 g fat (5.3 g saturated) 1.8 g salt	**Falafel Wrap**
284 calories 10.6 g fat (7.9 g saturated) 33.2 g sugar	**Chai Latte**

GUILTY PLEASURE

Palmine Biscuit

75 calories
4.5 g fat
(2.2 g saturated)

If you're craving something sweet with your coffee, this is your best bet. It beats pretty much every other biscuit on the Nero menu by around 150 calories. The only one that runs it close is the Almond Biscotti, at 147 calories. Beware of pretenders to the healthy eating throne such as the Organic Oat & Raisin Cookie. Sounds good doesn't it? But it actually has 248 calories.

MENU MAGIC

Nero has a whole range of healthy salads and soups, many of which clock in under the 200 calorie mark. In fact you can get the Organic Sundried Tomato & Basil Soup with a Cappuccino for afterwards and your entire lunch will come in at less than 200 calories. Add a ciabatta roll to soak up the soup and you're still only looking at 346 calories in total. Stirring stuff.

Costa

That quick trip to the coffee shop for a snack could see you downing nearly half your recommended daily calories—particularly if your trip happens to involve one of Costa's Cream Coolers. Food wise, however, it does offer a reasonable range of sandwiches, many of which are under 450 calories, and with extensive nutritional information published online it's easy to find out if you should think about switching your usual order.

SURVIVAL STRATEGY

Order a healthy drink, not an unhealthy one with skimmed milk. The skimmed Mocha Flake With Cream still has 423 calories.

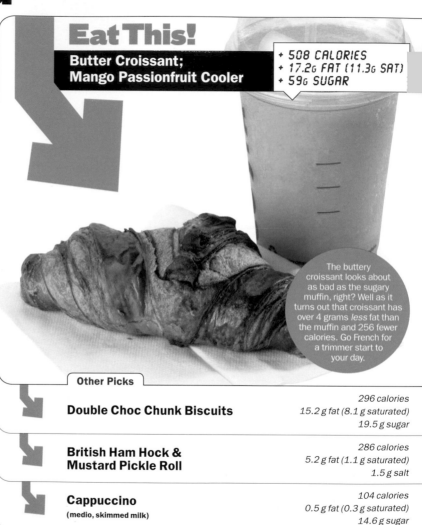

Eat This!

Butter Croissant; Mango Passionfruit Cooler

+ 508 CALORIES
+ 17.2G FAT (11.3G SAT)
+ 59G SUGAR

The buttery croissant looks about as bad as the sugary muffin, right? Well as it turns out that croissant has over 4 grams *less* fat than the muffin and 256 fewer calories. Go French for a trimmer start to your day.

Other Picks

Double Choc Chunk Biscuits

296 calories
15.2 g fat (8.1 g saturated)
19.5 g sugar

British Ham Hock & Mustard Pickle Roll

286 calories
5.2 g fat (1.1 g saturated)
1.5 g salt

Cappuccino
(medio, skimmed milk)

104 calories
0.5 g fat (0.3 g saturated)
14.6 g sugar

Not That!

Lemon and Poppyseed Muffin; Strawberry Cream Cooler

+ 1176 CALORIES
+ 43.8G FAT (12.5G SAT)
+ 123.7G SUGAR

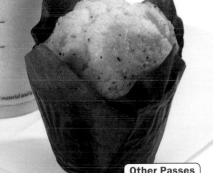

Costa's cold drinks range is a minefield. This creamy delight hides 644 calories. Think that you might be sidestepping the sugar in the fruity version? Sorry, this has 34 grams more of the white stuff than the Mango.

WEIGHT-GAIN BOMB
All Day Breakfast Roll

663 calories
33.6 g fat
(9.2 g saturated)

This is by far the unhealthiest sandwich on Costa's menu. It has nearly twice the calories of its breakfast counterpart the Egg & Mushroom Roll. It may be an all day breakfast, but have it every day and you'll regret it for years to come.

MENU MAGIC

Look past the muffins and pastries and make Costa's Strawberry & Granola Yogurt the centerpiece of your breakfast. Granola often gets a bad rap for being sugary, but here you get away with a modest 18.2 grams. Order some tropical fruit sticks and an Americano on the side. All told, your damage will come in under 370 calories—that's about 300 fewer than the All Day Breakfast Roll.

Other Passes

610 calories
29.2 g fat (6.2 g saturated)
64.2 g sugar

Coffee & Walnut Cake

528 calories
17 g fat (7.5 g saturated)
2.2 g salt

British Chicken & Chorizo Panini

502 calories
27.2 g fat (17 g saturated)
45.4 g sugar

Mocha Flake With Cream
(medio, full-fat milk)

Domino's

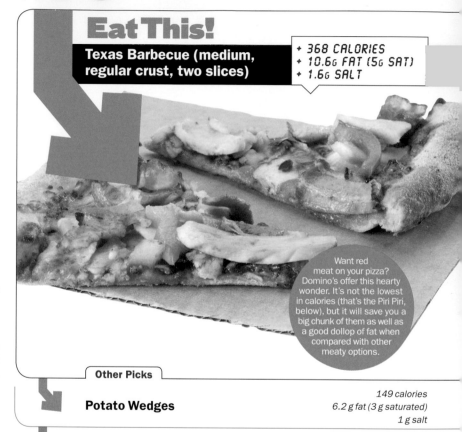

Domino's has some extremely calorific options on its menu, mainly involving meatballs. However, it does manage to make a cheese and tomato pizza that, unlike those from some other chains, isn't completely smothered in cheese, so works out being a sensible option. Of course, the less said about the Double Decadence and Dominator bases on offer, the better.

SURVIVAL STRATEGY

The problem with pizza is it's tempting to eat the whole thing. Don't. Instead treat it as a main to share and order a side to go with it. Domino's potato wedges have 311 fewer calories than a portion of large fries at McDonald's.

Eat This!

Texas Barbecue (medium, regular crust, two slices)

+ 368 CALORIES
+ 10.6G FAT (5G SAT)
+ 1.6G SALT

Want red meat on your pizza? Domino's offer this hearty wonder. It's not the lowest in calories (that's the Piri Piri, below), but it will save you a big chunk of them as well as a good dollop of fat when compared with other meaty options.

Other Picks

Potato Wedges

149 calories
6.2 g fat (3 g saturated)
1 g salt

Vegetarian Supreme Sub

468 calories
13.6 g fat (7.2 g saturated)
2.5 g salt

Piri Piri Pizza
(medium thin crust, one slice)

119 calories
5.6 g fat (2.2 g saturated)
0.6 g salt

Not That!

Meatball Mayhem (medium, regular crust, two slices)

+ 524 CALORIES
+ 19.4G FAT (8.1G SAT)
+ 2.8G SALT

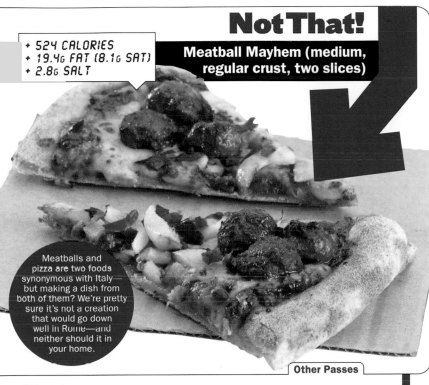

Meatballs and pizza are two foods synonymous with Italy—but making a dish from both of them? We're pretty sure it's not a creation that would go down well in Rome—and neither should it in your home.

ALL THIS

Two slices of a small, regular crust Cheese & Tomato Pizza, one portion each of Chicken Kickers and Potato Wedges and two Domino's Cookies

OR

THAT

Meateor Personal Pizza
815 calories

Other Passes

251 calories
15.3 g fat (6.7 g saturated)
1.5 g salt

Garlic Mozzarella Sticks

565 calories
28.2 g fat (15 g saturated)
3.5 g salt

Tuna Melt Sub

341 calories
13.8 g fat (5.1 g saturated)
1.4 g salt

Domnio's Meateor
(large Dominator base, one slice)

77

Eat

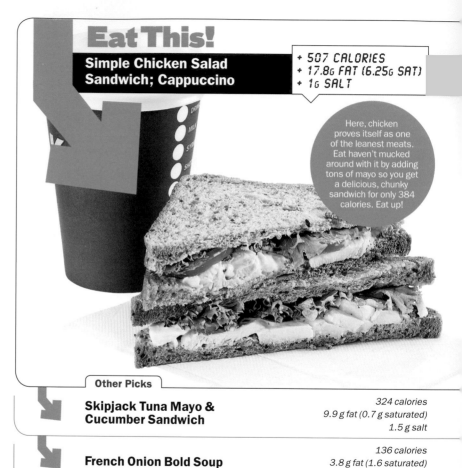

This chain has a shop on virtually every corner in London, and has branched out to major cities and airports nationwide. Their range is diverse with drinks, soups, salads and even pies. Unsurprisingly the pie range is pretty much out of bounds when it comes to healthy eating. Nevertheless there are plenty of decent options elsewhere on the menu, if you know where to look...

SURVIVAL STRATEGY

Eat has a big range of porridge. Eat it plain for a super-healthy and filling start to your day (add banana for only 20 extra calories in a small pot). At lunch look out for super-lean chicken dishes but avoid anything with carb-heavy noodles.

Eat This!

Simple Chicken Salad Sandwich; Cappuccino

+ 507 CALORIES
+ 17.8G FAT (6.25G SAT)
+ 1G SALT

Here, chicken proves itself as one of the leanest meats. Eat haven't mucked around with it by adding tons of mayo so you get a delicious, chunky sandwich for only 384 calories. Eat up!

Other Picks

Skipjack Tuna Mayo & Cucumber Sandwich
324 calories
9.9 g fat (0.7 g saturated)
1.5 g salt

French Onion Bold Soup
136 calories
3.8 g fat (1.6 saturated)
2.5 g salt

Tandoori Chicken, Mango & Rice Salad
244 calories
5.7 g fat (2 g saturated)
1.6 g salt

Not That!

Mature Cheddar & Real Ale Pickle Sandwich; Chai Latte

- **1044 CALORIES**
- **44.8G FAT (21.6G SAT)**
- **2.5G SALT**

The lesson to learn from the innocent looking sandwich? Cheese can be hazardous to your waistline... beer in your pickle even more so. This has around 250 more calories than the Simple Chicken. That Chai Latte is 408.

Other Passes

580 calories
28.9 g fat (8 g saturated)
3.3 g salt

Ham & Free Range Egg

456 calories
1.5 g fat (0.3 g saturated)
2.4 g salt

Old Fashioned Chicken and Egg Noodles Bold Soup

413 calories
13.7 g fat (2.6 g saturated)
2.3 g salt

Spicy Crayfish Noodle Salad

Greggs

Renowned for being one of the best value sandwich shops in the UK. Unfortunately good value doesn't always mean good for you. A lot of the menu is high in fat and as they don't publish a saturated fat breakdown, or sugar content for that matter, it can be tricky to sidestep the bad stuff. At least their drinks menu is simple, though, no Triple-Mocha Chai Gingerbread Lattes here.

SURVIVAL STRATEGY

Keep a wary eye out for Greggs' pastries. They sneak in on both the sweet and savoury sides of the menu adding who knows how much saturated fat to your meal. If you must indulge go for the smaller portions such as the Toffee Yum Yum.

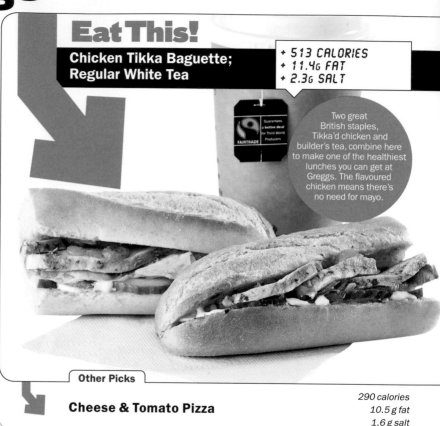

Eat This!

**Chicken Tikka Baguette;
Regular White Tea**

+ 513 CALORIES
+ 11.4G FAT
+ 2.3G SALT

FAIRTRADE
Guarantees a better deal for Third World Producers

Two great British staples, Tikka'd chicken and builder's tea, combine here to make one of the healthiest lunches you can get at Greggs. The flavoured chicken means there's no need for mayo.

Other Picks

Cheese & Tomato Pizza

290 calories
10.5 g fat
1.6 g salt

Ham Salad Oval Bite

320 calories
11.5 g fat
1.3 g salt

Mixed Berry and Granola Yoghurt

230 calories
7.5 g fat
30.5 carbohydrate

Not That!

**Chicken Club Baguette;
Regular Latte**

- **+ 870 CALORIES**
- **+ 33.8G FAT**
- **+ 2.4G SALT**

You'll pay for joining the Greggs club with nearly 200 extra calories over the Tikka version. And all that mayo actually means less meat: there's only a couple of grams more protein here, despite the bacon.

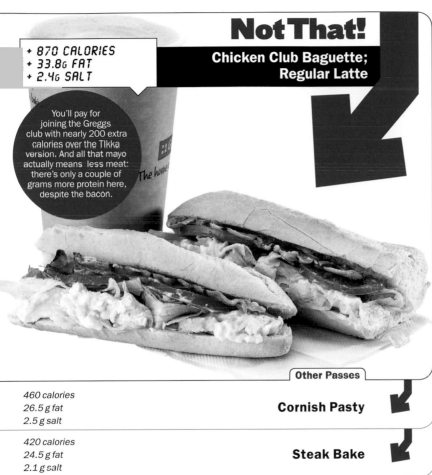

The home

Other Passes

460 calories 26.5 g fat 2.5 g salt	**Cornish Pasty**
420 calories 24.5 g fat 2.1 g salt	**Steak Bake**
570 calories 31 g fat 65 g carbohydrate	**Triple Chocolate Muffin**

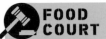

FOOD COURT

THE CRIME
Classic BLT with Sweetcure Bacon
(550 calories)

THE PUNISHMENT
An hour of running at 5mph
(12 minute miles)

11

The number of menu items made with pastry

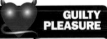

GUILTY PLEASURE

Toffee Yum Yum

290 calories
16.5 g fat
31.5 g carbohydrate

If you're sweet tooth is getting the better of you reach for one of these doughnut twists. The toffee flavoured version has 50 fewer calories than the regular one. It packs in a lot of sugar and fat for such a small portion (it's only 75g) but it's still the best item on the sweet menu. Just make sure you only have one.

KFC

The Colonel has really cleaned up his act recently by introducing 'Brazer' chicken done on the grill, rather than fried. There is a problem with this, however: you can't get it in all branches. One out of three KFCs that we tried in central London were able to deliver a Brazer Burger. One didn't have a grill and a second did have a grill but it was broken. Still, at least we burned extra calories walking to the third.

SURVIVAL STRATEGY

Go for the Brazer chicken whenever you can, otherwise you're at the mercy of the fatty, fried variety. And be imaginative with sides (hint: fries are the worst option).

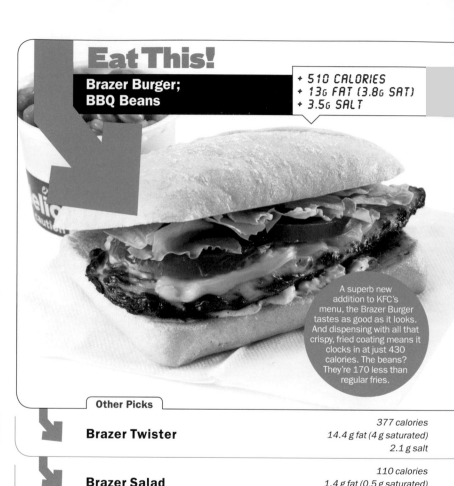

Eat This!

Brazer Burger; BBQ Beans

+ 510 CALORIES
+ 13G FAT (3.8G SAT)
+ 3.5G SALT

A superb new addition to KFC's menu, the Brazer Burger tastes as good as it looks. And dispensing with all that crispy, fried coating means it clocks in at just 430 calories. The beans? They're 170 less than regular fries.

Other Picks

Brazer Twister

377 calories
14.4 g fat (4 g saturated)
2.1 g salt

Brazer Salad

110 calories
1.4 g fat (0.5 g saturated)
1.2 g salt

Avalanche

173 calories
7.6 g fat (4.5 g saturated)
18.2 g sugar

Not That!

Fillet Tower Burger; Regular Fries

+ *896 CALORIES*
+ *43G FAT (10G SAT)*
+ *4G SALT*

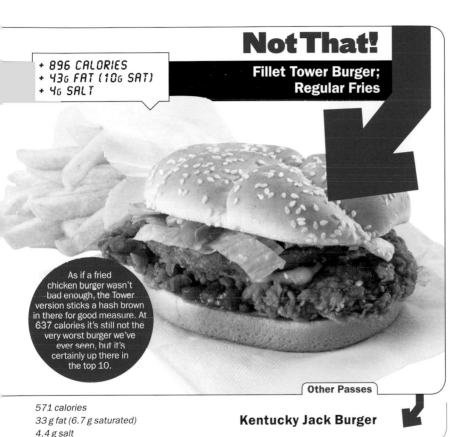

As if a fried chicken burger wasn't bad enough, the Tower version sticks a hash brown in there for good measure. At 637 calories it's still not the very worst burger we've ever seen, but it's certainly up there in the top 10.

WEIGHT-GAIN BOMB
Big Daddy Burger

674 calories
65.8 g fat
(14.5 g saturated)
6.6 g salt

With more salt than you should consume in a day, this burger is the single worst item on the KFC menu. It also has nearly all the Guideline Daily Amount of fat for one day and three quarters of your saturated fat allowance. The wonder is that, with all that bad stuff, it still comes in under 700 calories.

SMART SIDES

One of the best things about the KFC menu is that there are a few alternatives to fries with your burger. You can skip the huge calorie and fat count (379 calories and 18.9 grams of fat in large fries) by ordering one of these little wonders...

YOUR BEST BETS
Corn Cobette
148 calories, 8.4 g fat

BBQ Beans, Regular
88 calories, 0.6 g fat

Coleslaw, Regular
145 calories, 12.4 g fat

Other Passes

571 calories *33 g fat (6.7 g saturated)* *4.4 g salt*	**Kentucky Jack Burger**
307 calories *14.3 g fat (3 g saturated)* *2.4 g salt*	**Zinger Salad**
387 calories *13.2 g fat (7 g saturated)* *42.3 g sugar*	**Krushems Strawberry Shortcake**

McDonald's

The golden arches are shaking off their reputation as the gateway to weight gain. Their entire menu has calorie counts clearly displayed alongside each item and there also plenty of healthy options. Some obvious, like porridge for breakfast, others more surprising: who would've thought, for example that chicken nuggets would be better for you than fries?

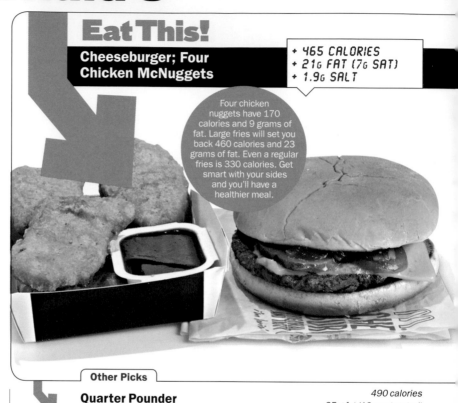

Eat This!

Cheeseburger; Four Chicken McNuggets

+ 465 CALORIES
+ 21G FAT (7G SAT)
+ 1.9G SALT

Four chicken nuggets have 170 calories and 9 grams of fat. Large fries will set you back 460 calories and 23 grams of fat. Even a regular fries is 330 calories. Get smart with your sides and you'll have a healthier meal.

Other Picks

Quarter Pounder With Cheese

490 calories
25 g fat (13 g saturated)
2.2 g salt

Oatso Simple with Apple & Berry Compote

225 calories
5 g fat (2 g saturated)
0.3g salt

Grilled Chicken & Bacon Salad

165 calories
5 g fat (2 g saturated)
1.1 g salt

Not That!

Sweet Chilli Crispy Chicken Wrap; Large French Fries

+ 920 CALORIES
+ 41ɢ FAT (5ɢ SAT)
+ 2.9ɢ SALT

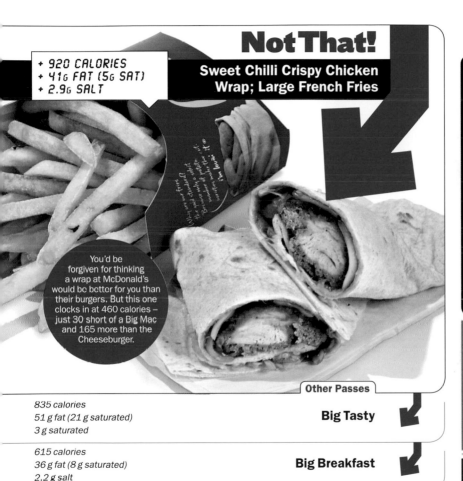

You'd be forgiven for thinking a wrap at McDonald's would be better for you than their burgers. But this one clocks in at 460 calories – just 30 short of a Big Mac and 165 more than the Cheeseburger.

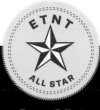

ETNT ALL STAR

Bacon & Egg McMuffin

345 calories
10 g fat
(6 g saturated)
1.4 g salt

Other breakfast sandwiches come and go, but the McMuffin never fails to deliver a crucial punch of protein (19 grams) during the morning hours. Given its status as one of the battle-tested veterans of the industry, the Bacon & Egg McMuffin would make your starting lineup in the Fast-Food All-Star Game.

ALL THIS

Bacon & Egg McMuffin, Oastso Simple with Apple & Berry Compote, Fruit Bag
612 calories

THAT

Big Breakfast
615 calories

Other Passes

835 calories 51 g fat (21 g saturated) 3 g saturated	**Big Tasty**
615 calories 36 g fat (8 g saturated) 2.2 g salt	**Big Breakfast**
325 calories 15 g fat (3 g saturated) 1.6 g salt	**Crispy Chicken & Bacon Salad**

Pret a Manger

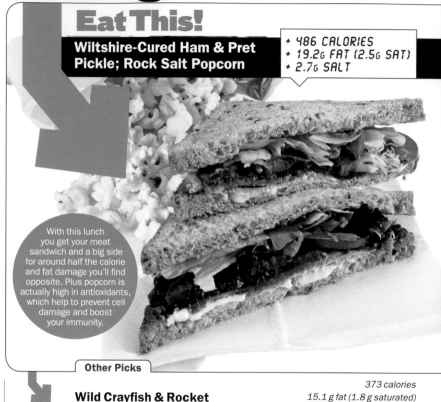

The UK's biggest sandwich chain now makes healthy eating easier with calorie counts alongside each product. They've also booted out fat in recent years with Pret yogurt dressing as an alternative to mayo. Even so, sometimes they don't hold back on the fillings, so it pays to check: a Ham & Egg Bloomer has 100 more calories than a Chicken, Ham & Cheese Club.

SURVIVAL STRATEGY

The soup range is almost all good with nearly everything under 300 calories, just keep a wary eye on for the odd 400+ curve ball like the Lentil & Coconut Dahl. Salads are also excellent, especially if you leave off the dressing.

Eat This!

Wiltshire-Cured Ham & Pret Pickle; Rock Salt Popcorn

+ 486 CALORIES
+ 19.2G FAT (2.5G SAT)
+ 2.7G SALT

With this lunch you get your meat sandwich and a big side for around half the calorie and fat damage you'll find opposite. Plus popcorn is actually high in antioxidants, which help to prevent cell damage and boost your immunity.

Other Picks

Wild Crayfish & Rocket
373 calories
15.1 g fat (1.8 g saturated)
1.9 g salt

Scottish Smoked Salmon
348 calories
11.5 g fat (6 g saturated)
2.6 g salt

Beef, Ale & Barley Soup
230 calories
6.7 g fat (0.7 g saturated)
1.4 g salt

Not That!

**All Day Breakfast;
Curry Lime Crisps**

+ 869 CALORIES
+ 51.4G FAT (10.9G SAT)
+ 3.3G SALT

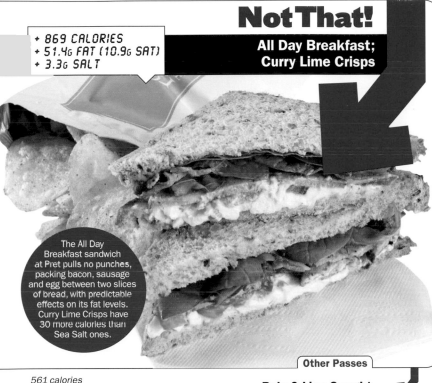

The All Day Breakfast sandwich at Pret pulls no punches, packing bacon, sausage and egg between two slices of bread, with predictable effects on its fat levels. Curry Lime Crisps have 30 more calories than Sea Salt ones.

Other Passes

561 calories
26..5 g fat (2.3 g saturated)
2.4g salt

**Pole & Line Caught
Tuna & Rocket Bloomer**

599 calories
25.7 g fat (4.7 g saturated)
3.4 g salt

Classic Ham & Eggs Bloomer

418 calories
17.4 g fat (11.5 g saturated)
2.3 g salt

Lentil & Coconut Dhal Soup

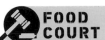

FOOD COURT

**THE CRIME
Pret Chocolate Brownie**
(369 calories)

**THE PUNISHMENT
An hour and a half walking on pavements**

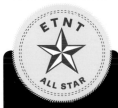

ETNT
ALL STAR

**Pole & Line Caught
Tuna Nicoise Salad**

138 calories
3.8 g fat
(1.4 g saturated)
0.9 g salt

This star player could be the saviour of your lunch hour. As well as the tuna, this salad includes Charlotte potatoes, free-range egg, green beans, tomatoes and red onion. Leave off the little pot of French dressing and you'll get all this for less than 140 calories. Plus there's less than 1 gram of salt, nearly 3 grams of fibre and a hefty 18.8 gram hit of protein. Probably the best salad in Britain.

Starbucks

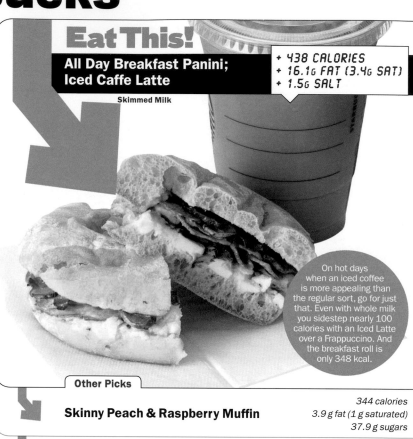

Starbucks' signature line of drinks typically involves injecting massive loads of sugary syrup and milk into an espresso, making 500-calorie concoctions too common for comfort. Plus, its baked good selection is a vortex of refined carbs. That said, Starbucks has bolstered its menu with porridge, healthy snacks, and better sandwiches and wraps and now make specialty drinks with skimmed milk.

SURVIVAL STRATEGY

There's no beating a regular cup of joe or unsweetened tea, but if you need a specialty fix, stick with fat-free milk, sugar-free syrup, and no whipped cream.

Eat This!

All Day Breakfast Panini; Iced Caffe Latte

Skimmed Milk

+ 438 CALORIES
+ 16.1G FAT (3.4G SAT)
+ 1.5G SALT

On hot days when an iced coffee is more appealing than the regular sort, go for just that. Even with whole milk you sidestep nearly 100 calories with an Iced Latte over a Frappuccino. And the breakfast roll is only 348 kcal.

Other Picks

Skinny Peach & Raspberry Muffin
344 calories
3.9 g fat (1 g saturated)
37.9 g sugars

Caffe Latte
Grande, Semi-Skimmed Milk
188 calories
7 g fat (4.4 g saturated)
16.5 g sugars

Free Range Egg Mayo Sandwich
372 calories
15.1 g fat (2.6 g saturated)
1 g salt

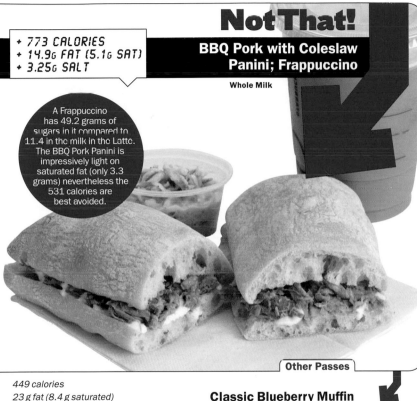

+ **773 CALORIES**
+ **14.9G FAT (5.1G SAT)**
+ **3.25G SALT**

Not That!

BBQ Pork with Coleslaw Panini; Frappuccino

Whole Milk

A Frappuccino has 49.2 grams of sugars in it compared to 11.4 in the milk in the Latte. The BBQ Pork Panini is impressively light on saturated fat (only 3.3 grams) nevertheless the 531 calories are best avoided.

Other Passes

449 calories
23 g fat (8.4 g saturated)
29.5 g sugars

Classic Blueberry Muffin

424 calories
12.9 g fat (8.8 g saturated)
59.9 g sugars

White Chocolate Mocha With Cream
Grande, Skimmed Milk

547 calories
24.2 g fat (13.3 g saturated)
2.25 g salt

Brie & Caramelised Onion Panini

CALORIE-CUTTING LINGO

● **Hold the whip:** Cuts the cream and saves you anywhere from 50 to 110 calories

● **Sugar-free syrup:** Use instead of regular syrup and save up to 150 calories a drink

● **Skinny:** Your drink will be made with sugar-free syrup and skimmed milk

Subway

In 2011 Subway overtook McDonald's as the world's largest restaurant chain. They usually beat the golden arches in the health stakes as well. Their range of low-fat subs and salads is particularly impressive, but don't fall into the trap of thinking that just because it comes in a baguette that it's healthy. It's amazing how much you can get in between two bits of bread in the name of breakfast.

SURVIVAL STRATEGY

Don't (a) drown your lunch in extra dressing (b) choose flavoured bread or (c) think wraps are a healthier option – they have nearly 150 extra caloires compared to a normal 6" sub.

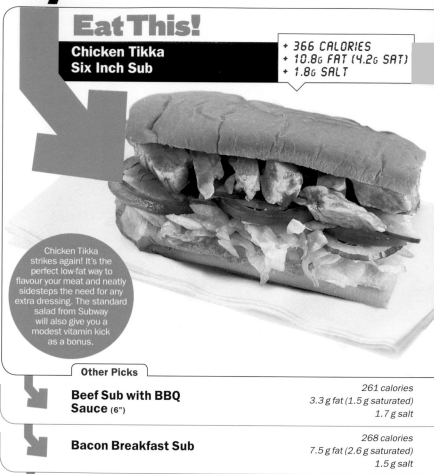

Eat This!

Chicken Tikka Six Inch Sub

+ 366 CALORIES
+ 10.8G FAT (4.2G SAT)
+ 1.8G SALT

Chicken Tikka strikes again! It's the perfect low-fat way to flavour your meat and neatly sidesteps the need for any extra dressing. The standard salad from Subway will also give you a modest vitamin kick as a bonus.

Other Picks

Beef Sub with BBQ Sauce (6")

261 calories
3.3 g fat (1.5 g saturated)
1.7 g salt

Bacon Breakfast Sub

268 calories
7.5 g fat (2.6 g saturated)
1.5 g salt

Veggie Delight Salad

52 calories
1 g fat (0.2 g saturated)
0.2 g salt

Not That!

Chicken & Bacon Six Inch Sub with Ranch Dressing

+ 540 CALORIES
+ 24.6G FAT (8.1G SAT)
+ 3.4G SALT

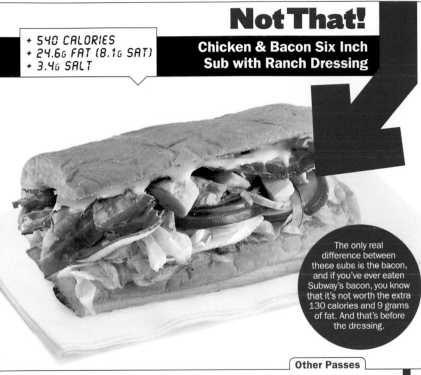

The only real difference between these subs is the bacon, and if you've ever eaten Subway's bacon, you know that it's not worth the extra 130 calories and 9 grams of fat. And that's before the dressing.

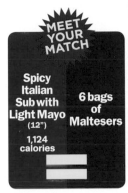

MEET YOUR MATCH

Spicy Italian Sub with Light Mayo (12")

1,124 calories

6 bags of Maltesers

11

The number of 6-inch subs with fewer than 350 calories

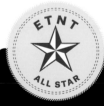

ETNT ALL STAR

Subway Club (6")

**298 calories
4.1g fat
(1.5g saturated)**

Normally the word 'club' is one to steer clear of in sandwiches. But at Subway the meat's lean the fat count stays low.

Other Passes

599 calories
29.9 g fat (9.7 g saturated)
3.7 g salt

Meatball Marinara Sub with Chipolte Southwest Sauce (6")

513 calories
24.7 g fat (8.6 g saturated)
2.9 g salt

Mega Breakfast Sub (6")

201 calories
3.4 g fat (0.7 g saturated)
1.7 g salt

Sweet Onion Chicken Teriyaki Salad

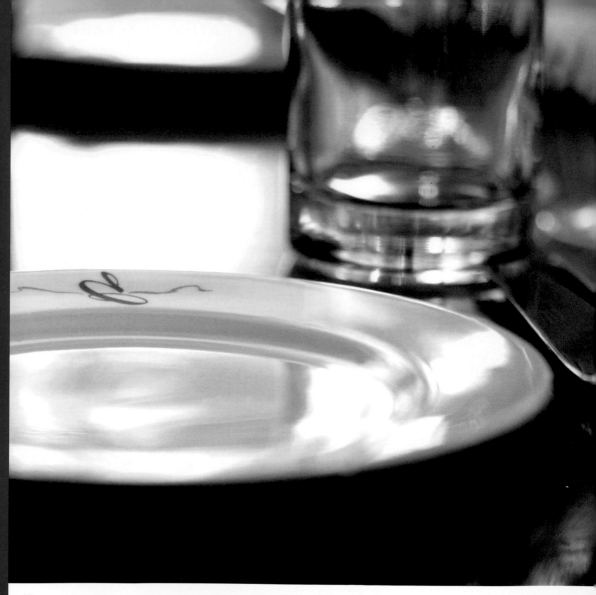

When you go out for a sit-down meal nutrition might not be the first thing on your mind. But it pays to brush up, because waistline destroyers lurk in unexpected places on some menus

Restaurants

Bella Italia

Like sister restaurant Café Rouge (overleaf), Bella Italia only publishes calorie counts, but promises more nutritional info is in the pipeline. We're hoping it'll be ready for the next edition of *Eat This, Not That*. It currently highlights dishes under 600 calories with a symbol on its menu. As does Café Rouge. These days both chains are owned by the same company, Tragus, which is moving in the right direction nutrition wise.

SURVIVAL STRATEGY

Stick to the sub-600 items on the menu and you can't go too far wrong. Avoid the meaty breakfast options and go veggie to save on calories.

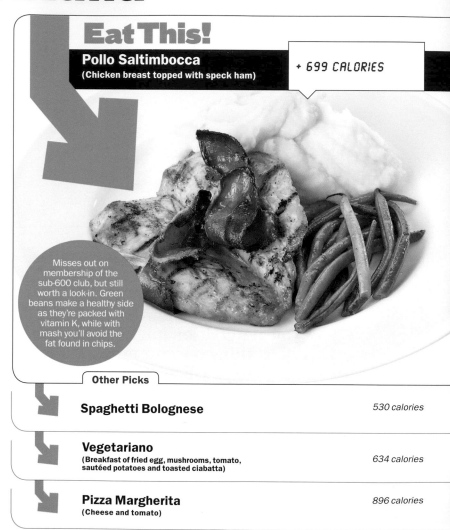

Eat This!

Pollo Saltimbocca
(Chicken breast topped with speck ham)

+ 699 CALORIES

Misses out on membership of the sub-600 club, but still worth a look-in. Green beans make a healthy side as they're packed with vitamin K, while with mash you'll avoid the fat found in chips.

Other Picks

Spaghetti Bolognese

530 calories

Vegetariano
(Breakfast of fried egg, mushrooms, tomato, sautéed potatoes and toasted ciabatta)

634 calories

Pizza Margherita
(Cheese and tomato)

896 calories

Not That!

Burger Americano

+ 1508 CALORIES

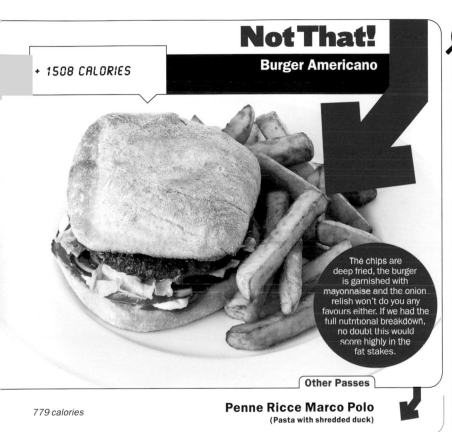

The chips are deep fried, the burger is garnished with mayonnaise and the onion relish won't do you any favours either. If we had the full nutritional breakdown, no doubt this would score highly in the fat stakes.

Other Passes

779 calories	**Penne Ricce Marco Polo** (Pasta with shredded duck)	
908 calories	**Bacon and Egg Panini**	
1,340 calories	**Pizza Pesto Rosso E Verdure** (Peppers, onions, olives, tomatoes, mushrooms, red pesto, mascarpone and mozzarella)	

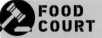

FOOD COURT

THE CRIME
Inglese
Full English breakfast of scrambled eggs, bacon, sausage, mushroom, tomato, sautéed potatoes, toasted ciabatta
(1,286 calories)

THE PUNISHMENT
2 hours 10 minutes doing crunches

TOPPING DECODER
Top 10 worst extras to add to your pizza

1. **MARSCAPONE**
245 calories

2. **GREEN PESTO**
198 calories

3. **SALSA VERDE**
165 calories

4. **EGG**
164 calories

5. **RED PESTO**
140 calories

6. **HAM PIECES**
133 calories

7. **PEPPERONI**
105 calories

8. **DUCK**
95 calories

9. **SPRING ONION**
73 calories

10. **ROAST COURGETTES**
72 calories

Café Rouge

As with Bella Italia (previous page), Café Rouge only publishes calorie counts but says a full nutritional breakdown is on the way—putting it firmly in the growing club of restaurants which care about healthy eating. Pressure is on the dwindling number of chains which (somewhat suspiciously) find it unnecessary to subject their food to nutritional analysis of any kind. Wagamama anyone...?

SURVIVAL STRATEGY

Like Bella Italia, there's a section of the menu that flags up all dishes containing under 600 calories. This means health-conscious diners will always have a variety of guilt-free options to chose from.

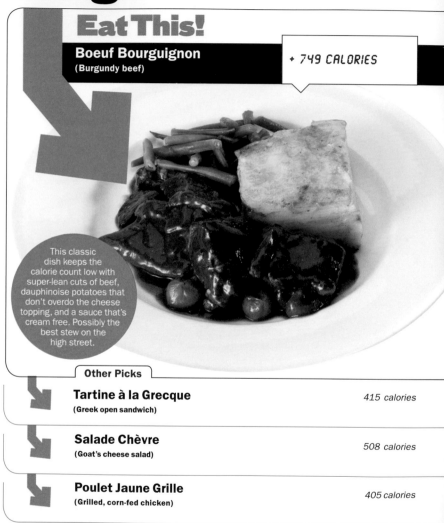

Eat This!

Boeuf Bourguignon
(Burgundy beef)

+ 749 CALORIES

This classic dish keeps the calorie count low with super-lean cuts of beef, dauphinoise potatoes that don't overdo the cheese topping, and a sauce that's cream free. Possibly the best stew on the high street.

Other Picks

Tartine à la Grecque
(Greek open sandwich)

415 calories

Salade Chèvre
(Goat's cheese salad)

508 calories

Poulet Jaune Grille
(Grilled, corn-fed chicken)

405 calories

Not That!

Salade Paysanne
(Farmer's salad)

+ 1101 CALORIES

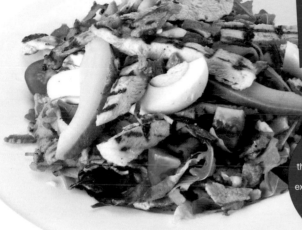

The chicken, bacon, avocado and egg all combine to bump the calorie count here up to way beyond what you'd expect from a salad. Even so we think that 'lemon and garlic' dressing still has a lot to answer for.

Other Passes

1,249 calories	**Baguette Rouge**
908 calories	**Saumon Nicoise** (Salmon salad)
1,067 calories	**Poulet Breton** (Brittany chicken)

WEIGHT-GAIN BOMB
Baguette Poulet
(chicken baguette)

1,204 calories

You might think that ordering a big chicken sandwich would be a reasonably safe bet. Not so at Café Rouge. It comes with fries, which don't have calories listed separately but appear to be worth at least 500 on top of any dish they're served with. Just for the record, six Chicken McNuggets and Regular Fries at McDonald's is 580 calories.

ALL THIS

Salade Entrecote
(steak salad)

Bouillabaisse
(fish stew)

Crème Brûlée
(cream pudding)

OR

THAT

Croque Saumon
(Salmon and cheese melt with fries and salad)

1,289 calories

Nando's

Nando's has changed the image of restaurant chicken in recent years. It proves that chuck doesn't have to be served fried, breaded or in a roll in order to be delicious. We also applaud the fact that it offers a whole range of tasty alternatives to chips, which is just as well really: its large Peri Peri Chips are probably the worst you can buy anywhere, clocking in at 1,074 calories with 44 g fat.

SURVIVAL STRATEGY

You're encouraged to eat more than you need, as two sides are included as a special deal with a lot of dishes. However, if you order just the dish and one regular side you'll be saving money as well as calories.

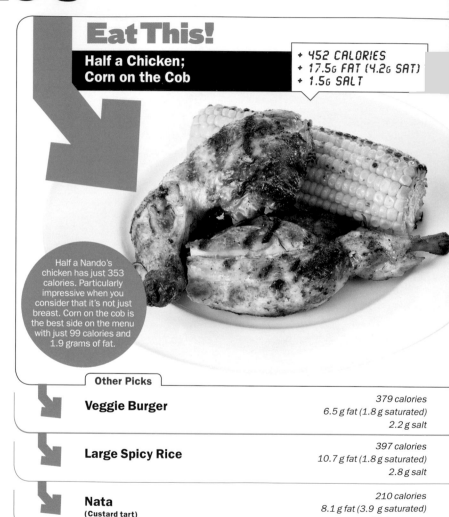

Eat This!

Half a Chicken; Corn on the Cob

+ 452 CALORIES
+ 17.5G FAT (4.2G SAT)
+ 1.5G SALT

Half a Nando's chicken has just 353 calories. Particularly impressive when you consider that it's not just breast. Corn on the cob is the best side on the menu with just 99 calories and 1.9 grams of fat.

Other Picks

Veggie Burger

379 calories
6.5 g fat (1.8 g saturated)
2.2 g salt

Large Spicy Rice

397 calories
10.7 g fat (1.8 g saturated)
2.8 g salt

Nata
(Custard tart)

210 calories
8.1 g fat (3.9 g saturated)
16.1 g sugars

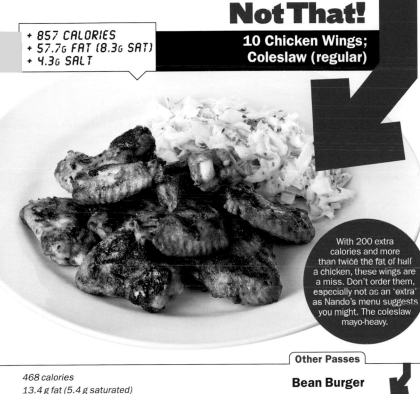

Not That!

**10 Chicken Wings;
Coleslaw (regular)**

+ *857 CALORIES*
+ *57.7G FAT (8.3G SAT)*
+ *4.3G SALT*

With 200 extra calories and more than twice the fat of half a chicken, these wings are a miss. Don't order them, especially not as an 'extra' as Nando's menu suggests you might. The coleslaw mayo-heavy.

SMART SIDES

Nando's has an excellent selection of sides. Here are the ones that should be within your sites. The creamy mash sneaks in as a better potato fix than those chips.

YOUR BEST BETS
Regular Creamy Mash
272 calories, 15.8 g fat

Mixed Leaf Salad
17 calories, 0.4 g fat

Ratatouille
185 calories, 13 g fat

Other Passes

468 calories
13.4 g fat (5.4 g saturated)
57 g sugars

Bean Burger

371 calories
24.8 g fat (3.2 g saturated)
2.3 g salt

Large Chips

726 calories
49.7 g fat (17.2 g saturated)
43.9 g salt

Carrot Cake

Pizza Express

Pizza has overtaken curry as the nation's favourite dish, with **90 percent of us eating it at least once a week.** And Pizza Express is among the favourite places to eat it. Although it looks like being the healthiest pizza chain in the country, it's unable to cement that claim, because it doesn't publish full nutritional information. Come on! It can't be that hard to give Pizza Hut and Domino's a run for their money.

SURVIVAL STRATEGY

Skip past anything with extra bread and go straight to the Leggera—a new part of the menu where all the pizzas are under 500 calories.

Eat This!

La Reine

+ 717 CALORIES

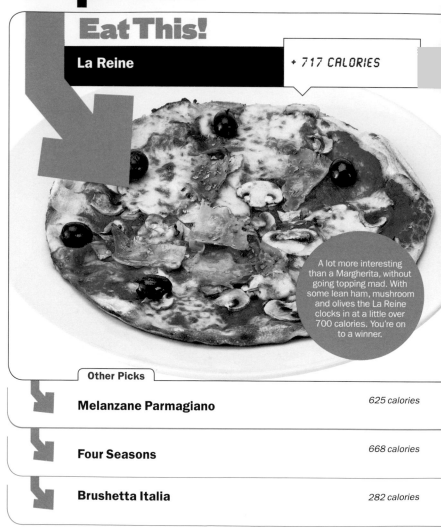

A lot more interesting than a Margherita, without going topping mad. With some lean ham, mushroom and olives the La Reine clocks in at a little over 700 calories. You're on to a winner.

Other Picks

Melanzane Parmagiano	*625 calories*
Four Seasons	*668 calories*
Brushetta Italia	*282 calories*

Not That!

Giardineria

+ 925 CALORIES

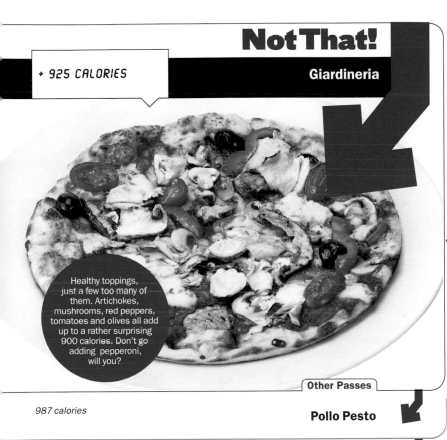

Healthy toppings, just a few too many of them. Artichokes, mushrooms, red peppers, tomatoes and olives all add up to a rather surprising 900 calories. Don't go adding pepperoni, will you?

Other Passes

987 calories   **Pollo Pesto**

920 calories   **Il Padrino**

534 calories   **Bruschetta con Funghi**

3

The number of pizzas over 1,000 calories: Calabrese, Etna and Salsicca Speziata (all Romana base)

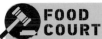

FOOD COURT

THE CRIME
Warm Vegetable and Goats Cheese Salad with Chicken
(909 calories)

THE PUNISHMENT
1 hours 45 minutes on a stair machine

 LITTLE TRICK

Pizza Express will make your pizza with less mozzarella or fatty meats if you ask your waiter.

Pizza Hut

The world's biggest pizza chain is renowned for making pizza in the American style: thick bases and tonnes of cheese. But it is possible to get a thin base and some fresh toppings. Nevertheless, Pizza Hut remains inordinately proud of its Stuffed Crust and Cheesy Bites bases. Apart from the health issues, why mess with centuries old Italian cuisine?

SURVIVAL STRATEGY

Always go for the Italian base and be wary of anything with extra pepperoni or cheese. And always share. Four slices of 14in pizza is a feast. Plus, when you're eating in you get unlimited salad on the side, so take advantage.

Eat This!

Farmhouse, Large Italian
(two slices)

+ 326 CALORIES
+ 15.8G FAT (6.6G SAT)
+ 2.6G SALT

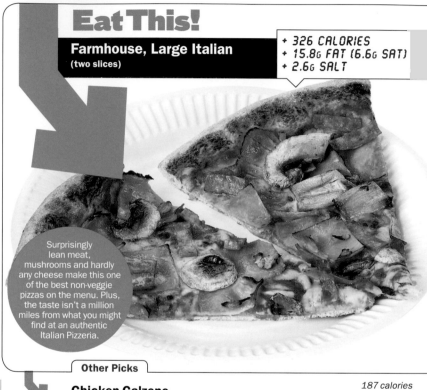

Surprisingly lean meat, mushrooms and hardly any cheese make this one of the best non-veggie pizzas on the menu. Plus, the taste isn't a million miles from what you might find at an authentic Italian Pizzeria.

Other Picks

Chicken Calzone

187 calories
5.3 g fat (2.5 g saturated)
1 g salt

Potato Skins, Cheese and Onion

406 calories
18.1 g fat (8.3 g saturated)
0.84 g salt

Chilli Twists

441 calories
13.1 g fat (1.8 g saturated)
3.27 g salt

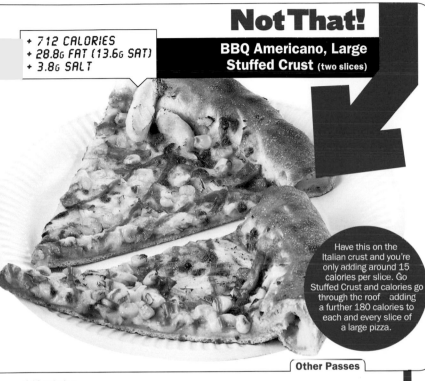

+ **712 CALORIES**
+ **28.8G FAT (13.6G SAT)**
+ **3.8G SALT**

Not That!

BBQ Americano, Large Stuffed Crust (two slices)

Have this on the Italian crust and you're only adding around 15 calories per slice. Go Stuffed Crust and calories go through the roof — adding a further 180 calories to each and every slice of a large pizza.

Other Passes

246 calories 10 g fat (4.1 g saturated) 1,120 mg sodium	**Meat Calzone**
554 calories 30 g fat (12 g saturated) 2.06 g salt	**Garlic Bread with Cheese**
832 calories 49.1 g fat (25.4 g saturated) 3.27g salt	**Salmon Pasta Bake**

BAD NEWS

Calorie Confusion

Pizza Hut includes some rudimentary calorie counts on its online menu. But the stats are at best confusing and at worst inaccurate. **Calories per slice only apply to the Regular Italian base,** a little disingenuous, but fine. Then the menu says calories will be more on a Pan, Stuffed Crust or Cheesy Bites base. It says to add 20 calories per slice for Pan and 60 per slice for the other two. This is roughly true if you're basing everything on its regular size. But wait, what's this? **Cheesy Bites doesn't come in regular size. Only large. So adding 60 calories won't nearly bridge the gap. Instead you should look at adding more like 180 calories per slice.** What it also fails to mention is you can actually upgrade any Italian base from regular to large for only around 5 calories per slice. Once you've done that bridging the gap to a large Pan will be around 120 calories and you'll be adding that 180 for a Stuffed Crust upgrade. Stuff that. One saving grace is that there is a full nutritional breakdown for all pizzas available to download. We'd prefer Pizza Hut to get it right on its menu, though.

Prezzo

The first Prezzo opened in central London in 2000, now the Italian chain has 150 restaurants across the UK. Despite its size, it manages to retain a fresh feel to dishes by regularly updating the menu: top chef Aldo Zilli created its VIPizzas. Prezzo has won a few awards, but it'll need to publish more than just the calorie count for its menu before winning an award from us.

SURVIVAL STRATEGY

There's an entire Light Options section of the menu, but salads are also excellent (all under 600 calories) as are the three grilled chicken dishes (not the sandwich). Be careful with the sides.

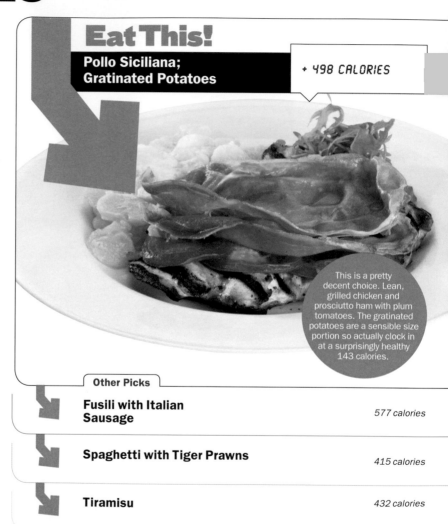

Eat This!

Pollo Siciliana; Gratinated Potatoes

+ 498 CALORIES

This is a pretty decent choice. Lean, grilled chicken and prosciutto ham with plum tomatoes. The gratinated potatoes are a sensible size portion so actually clock in at a surprisingly healthy 143 calories.

Other Picks

Fusili with Italian Sausage	*577 calories*
Spaghetti with Tiger Prawns	*415 calories*
Tiramisu	*432 calories*

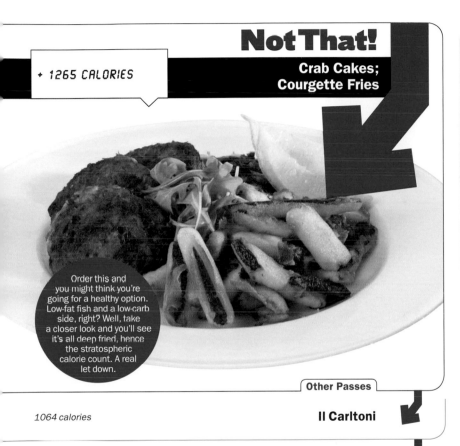

Not That!

Crab Cakes;
Courgette Fries

+ 1265 CALORIES

Order this and you might think you're going for a healthy option. Low-fat fish and a low-carb side, right? Well, take a closer look and you'll see it's all deep fried, hence the stratospheric calorie count. A real let down.

Other Passes

1064 calories	**Il Carltoni**
711 calories	**Tiger Prawn Risotto**
620 calories	**Milk Chocolate Fudge Cake**

ETNT ALL STAR

Chicken Caesar Salad
587 calories

This is one of those classic dishes that can easily creep up to the 1,000 calorie mark thanks to the Parmesan, croutons and fat-laden dressing. Prezzo keeps all this under control. Plus you can have it with prawns to save a further 87 calories. Or go veggie and you'll get a dish that's just 387 calories all told.

SMART SIDES

Skip courgette fries (568 calories!) you'll find a good range of side dishes at Prezzo. Even the House Fries are OK at 307 calories. But it gets better. This is our top 5:

Mixed salad
56 calories

Tomato & Red Onion Salad
87 calories

Gratinated Potatoes
143 calories

Rocket & Gran Padano Cheese Salad
193 calories

Caesar Side Salad
199 calories

Strada

Tragus, the owners of Bella Italia and Café Rouge, also own Strada. Health wise, the food varies from the surprisingly slimline to the unnecessarily calorie laden—and, once again, the menu has healthy options (under 600 calories) clearly marked. Strada has over 60 restaurants nationwide, bringing Tragus's total to over 200: it wields huge influence over what we eat when we're out.

SURVIVAL STRATEGY

Avoid the 'Pane' (bread) section on the menu. If you were to share the Cesto di Pane Misto with a friend and you'll both have 500 calories before you've even had a starter.

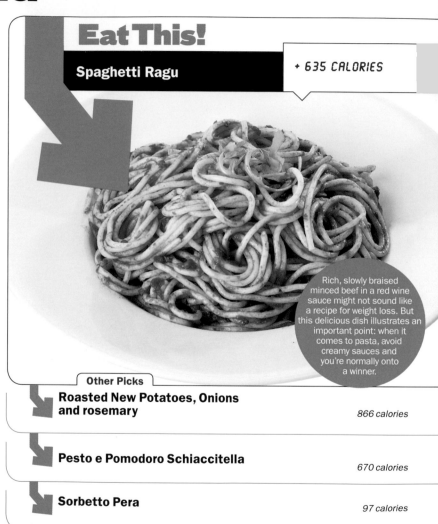

Eat This!

Spaghetti Ragu

+ 635 CALORIES

Rich, slowly braised minced beef in a red wine sauce might not sound like a recipe for weight loss. But this delicious dish illustrates an important point: when it comes to pasta, avoid creamy sauces and you're normally onto a winner.

Other Picks

Roasted New Potatoes, Onions and rosemary

866 calories

Pesto e Pomodoro Schiaccitella

670 calories

Sorbetto Pera

97 calories

Not That!

+ 1113 CALORIES

Rigatoni Speck

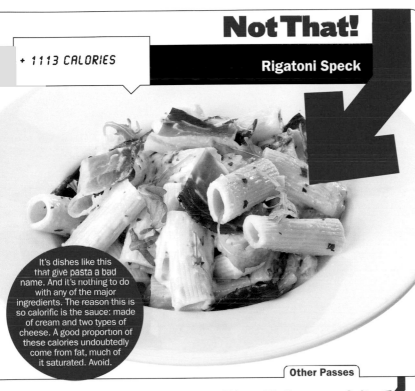

It's dishes like this that give pasta a bad name. And it's nothing to do with any of the major ingredients. The reason this is so calorific is the sauce: made of cream and two types of cheese. A good proportion of these calories undoubtedly come from fat, much of it saturated. Avoid.

Other Passes

Fries with Rosemary Salt
754 calories

Rustics Pizza
1,198 calories

Mousse al Ciocclato
866 calories

GUILTY PLEASURE

Gelato
179 to 277 calories

This Italian ice cream, contains less fat has more flavour and is easier on the waistline than normal. Whether Espresso or Pistachio, these cool delights are slightly healthier desserts.

MENU MAGIC

There are two fish dishes, Tegamiaccio (fish stew) and Tonno Nizzarda (seared tuna and bean salad), which for some reason aren't highlighted as being below 600 calories on the Strada menu, despite clocking in at 385 and 458 respectively. Go for either of these and you'll get a low-fat, protein packed feast.

FOOD COURT

THE CRIME
Bistecca Manzo
(10oz rib-eye with fries)
(1,187 calories)

THE PUNISHMENT
3 hours 45 minutes feeding cows on a farm

JD Wetherspoon

This chain of pubs offers cheap food, which is great for saving money, but not so great as its menu is awash with saturated fat: you get 121 percent of your RDA in a large breakfast. Not only that, its dishes regularly bust the 1,000 calorie mark, even in places you wouldn't expect, like the 1,023 calorie cheese, tomato and onion tart. Proof that you get what you pay for.

SURVIVAL STRATEGY

Avoid the saturated fat heavy meat, especially if it's fried. Even the 8oz sirloin (normally a lean cut) and chips has 28g, that's 143 percent of your daily amount. Its bacon sarnie will cost you a hefty 546kcal and 9.4 g saturated fat.

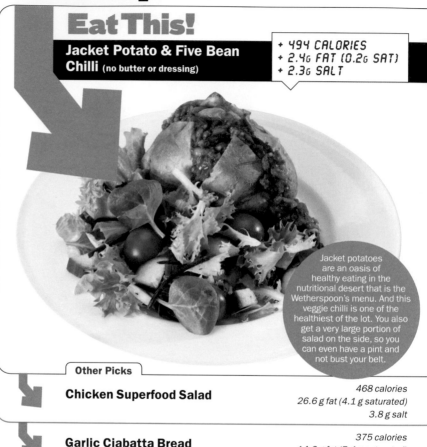

Eat This!

Jacket Potato & Five Bean Chilli (no butter or dressing)

+ 494 CALORIES
+ 2.4G FAT (0.2G SAT)
+ 2.3G SALT

Jacket potatoes are an oasis of healthy eating in the nutritional desert that is the Wetherspoon's menu. And this veggie chilli is one of the healthiest of the lot. You also get a very large portion of salad on the side, so you can even have a pint and not bust your belt.

Other Picks

Chicken Superfood Salad
468 calories
26.6 g fat (4.1 g saturated)
3.8 g salt

Garlic Ciabatta Bread
375 calories
14.6 g fat (7.4 g saturated)
1.4 g salt

Fresh Fruit and Yogurt
290 calories
1.9 g fat (1g saturated)
0 g salt

Not That!

Large Mixed Grill

- 1885 CALORIES
- 118G FAT (42G SAT)
- 6.8G SALT

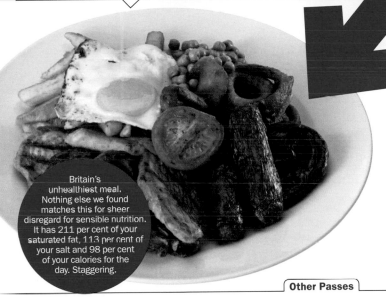

Britain's unhealthiest meal. Nothing else we found matches this for sheer disregard for sensible nutrition. It has 211 per cent of your saturated fat, 113 per cent of your salt and 98 per cent of your calories for the day. Staggering.

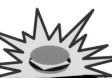

BURGER BOMB

Gourmet Beef Burger

1,828 calories
104g fat
(38.9g saturated)
8g salt

One for gluttons not gourmets, this whopping burger is almost as bad as the Large Mixed Grill. It comes loaded with two types of cheese, two bacon rashers, onion rings and a massive calorie count. Your body will not thank you.

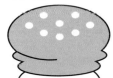

SALT LICK

GAMMON STEAK, EGG & CHIPS

9.9g salt
1,054 calories
58.8g fat
(15.2g saturated)

Never mind the thousand plus calories, this plate full has almost 10 g of salt. This is 165 percent of your guideline daily amount.

Other Passes

759 calories
52.9 g fat (17.4 g saturated)
1,590 mg sodium

Chicken Caesar Salad

752 calories
30.4 g fat (2.6 g saturated)
0.3 g salt

Bowl of Chips

809 calories
26.3 g fat (12.8 g saturated)
0.9 g salt

Belgian Waffles with Ice Cream

Yo Sushi

Few among us would enter Yo Sushi, grab a single bowl of Chicken Gyoza, munch down the 119-calorie dish and consider themselves well fed. It's all about combination cuisine, mixing your flavours to suit taste. So it's worth being aware that the wrong combination can be a recipe for disaster. With readily available nutritional information and easy portion control, Yo Sushi is a good bet if you choose wisely.

SURVIVAL STRATEGY

The simple way to eat well here is to limit the amount of dirty dishes you create. Three is enough for a balanced meal that will fill you up without putting strain on your innards.

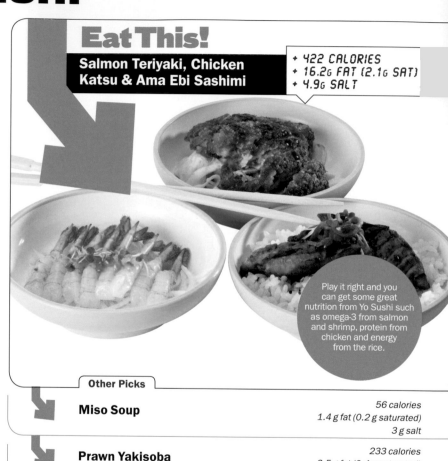

Eat This!

Salmon Teriyaki, Chicken Katsu & Ama Ebi Sashimi

+ 422 CALORIES
+ 16.2G FAT (2.1G SAT)
+ 4.9G SALT

Play it right and you can get some great nutrition from Yo Sushi such as omega-3 from salmon and shrimp, protein from chicken and energy from the rice.

Other Picks

Miso Soup
56 calories
1.4 g fat (0.2 g saturated)
3 g salt

Prawn Yakisoba
233 calories
3.5 g fat (0.4 g saturated)
5.2 g salt

Dorayaki
135 calories
1.3 g fat (0.5 g saturated)
8.9 g sugar

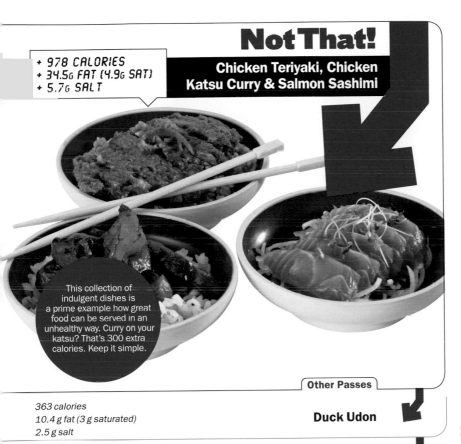

Not That!

Chicken Teriyaki, Chicken Katsu Curry & Salmon Sashimi

+ 978 CALORIES
+ 34.5G FAT (4.9G SAT)
+ 5.7G SALT

This collection of indulgent dishes is a prime example how great food can be served in an unhealthy way. Curry on your katsu? That's 300 extra calories. Keep it simple.

Other Passes

363 calories
10.4 g fat (3 g saturated)
2.5 g salt

Duck Udon

413 calories
7.8 g fat (1.3 g saturated)
3.6 g salt

Chicken Firecracker Rice

285 calories
8.2 g fat (4.2 g saturated)
3.6 g salt

Lemon Shortbread Cake

LITTLE TRICK

If you want to go seriously light, get the Miso Soup. At just 56 calories it's a little wonder.

111

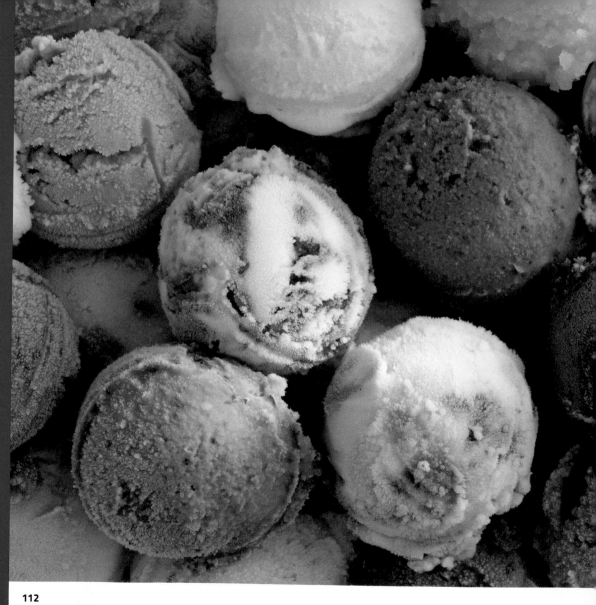

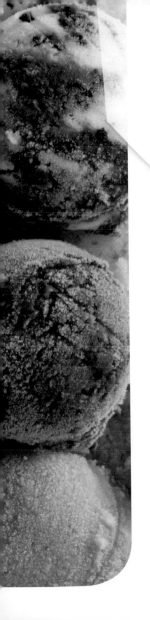

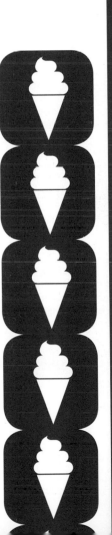

You've already decided to indulge your sweet tooth, but the question is how much is too much? This section has the answers you seek

Sweet Stuff

Baskin-Robbins

On their UK website Baskin-Robbins reveal how much fibre and salt is in their flavours... and that's it. Guess what? Every flavour is low in fibre and salt. But what about calories, fat and sugar? They do publish this information in the US. And, while not all flavours are the same, Baskin-Robbins confirmed, that for the ones that are, values will be similar. So we can at least give you some analysis here.

SURVIVAL STRATEGY

With choices such as yogurt, sherbet and sorbet, Baskin's lighter menu is the one bright spot in an otherwise darkly calorific place. Order the sugar cone instead of the waffle to save 160 calories.

Eat This!

2 Scoop Hot Fudge Sundae

+ 530 CALORIES
+ 29G FAT (19G SAT)
+ 51G SUGARS

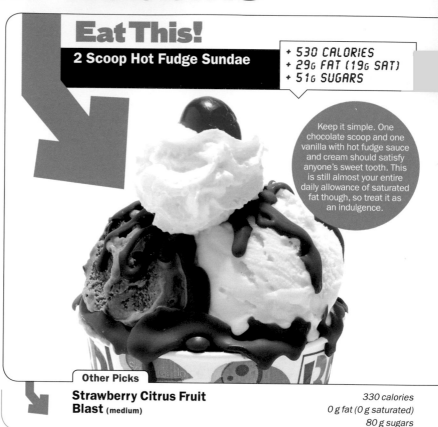

Keep it simple. One chocolate scoop and one vanilla with hot fudge sauce and cream should satisfy anyone's sweet tooth. This is still almost your entire daily allowance of saturated fat though, so treat it as an indulgence.

Other Picks

Strawberry Citrus Fruit Blast (medium)
330 calories
0 g fat (0 g saturated)
80 g sugars

Gold Medal Ribbon (1 scoop)
170 calories
8 g fat (5 g saturated)
19 g sugars

Cappuccino Blast (small)
280 calories
9 g fat (6 g saturated)
21 g sugars

114

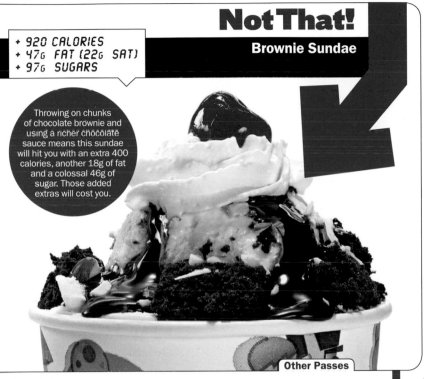

Not That!
Brownie Sundae

+ 920 CALORIES
+ 47G FAT (22G SAT)
+ 97G SUGARS

Throwing on chunks of chocolate brownie and using a richer chocolate sauce means this sundae will hit you with an extra 400 calories, another 18g of fat and a colossal 46g of sugar. Those added extras will cost you.

Other Passes

620 calories
2 g fat (0 g saturated)
144 g sugars

Wild Mango Smoothie
(medium)

200 calories
10 g fat (6 g saturated)
20 g sugars

Chocolate Chip Cookie Dough
(1 scoop)

670 calories
31 g fat (21 g saturated)
73 g sugars

Vanilla Shake
(small)

BAD NEWS
31° Below

These blended desserts all pack at least 600 calories—and most are closer to 1,000. In fact, the Fudge Brownie 31° Below contains 1,390 calories and 28 grams of saturated fat. That's 140% of your daily sat-fat allowance right there!

19

The Guinness World Record for the number of ice cream cones scooped in less than a minute, held by Baskin-Robbins employee Mitch Cohen

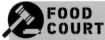

FOOD COURT

THE CRIME
Large Chocolate Chip Shake
(1,480 calories)

THE PUNISHMENT
Mop the floor for 6 hours

Ben & Jerry's

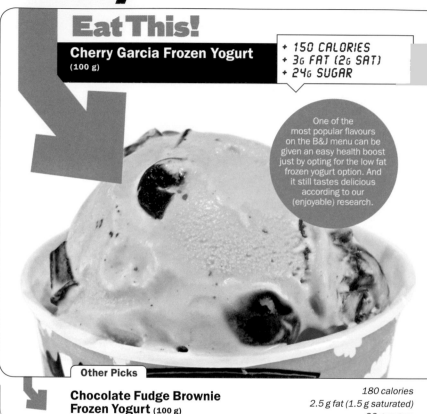

What sets B&J's apart from their competitors amounts to more than just an affinity for music festivals and green pastures. The shop also adheres to a lofty commitment to the quality and sources of its ingredients. All dairy is free from rBGH (recombinant bovine growth hormone) and the chocolate, vanilla, and coffee they use are all Fairtrade certified. From a strictly nutritional standpoint, though, it's still just an ice cream shop.

SURVIVAL STRATEGY

As with the Cherry Garcia, by choosing the low fat frozen yogurt option instead of ice cream you can save yourself 100 calories, 10g of fat and a lot of heart ache later in life.

Eat This!

Cherry Garcia Frozen Yogurt (100 g)

+ 150 CALORIES
+ 3G FAT (2G SAT)
+ 24G SUGAR

One of the most popular flavours on the B&J menu can be given an easy health boost just by opting for the low fat frozen yogurt option. And it still tastes delicious according to our (enjoyable) research.

Other Picks

Chocolate Fudge Brownie Frozen Yogurt (100 g)

180 calories
2.5 g fat (1.5 g saturated)
26 g sugars

Vanilla (100 g)

230 calories
15 g fat (10 g saturated)
20 g sugars

Baked Alaska (100 g)

260 calories
14 g fat (10 g saturated)
28 g sugars

Not That!

Chocolate Fudge Brownie
(100 g)

+ 250 CALORIES
+ 13G FAT (8G SAT)
+ 26G SUGAR

Another menu favourite, however, turns out to be one of the worst (though still overshadowed by the offending items listed below). Don't eat too much of this one, lest you end up with a bigger gut.

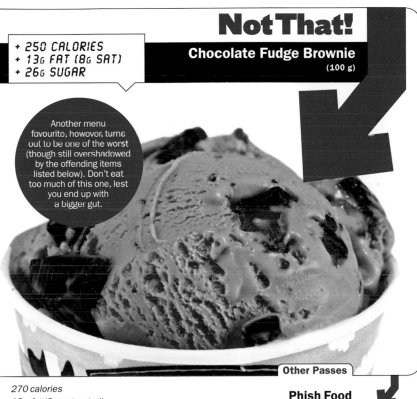

Other Passes

270 calories
13 g fat (9 g saturated)
32 g sugars

Phish Food
(100 g)

280 calories
16 g fat (11 g saturated)
29 g sugars

Caramel Chew Chew
(100 g)

280 calories
17 g fat (10 g saturated)
27 g sugars

Chunky Monkey
(100 g)

ICE CREAM EQUATIONS

SORBET
Water + sugar + fruit puree =
100 calories per serving for any and all flavours

FROZEN YOGURT
Skimmed milk + water + sugar + flavourings (cookie dough, raspberry puree, and so on) =
130 to 180 calories per serving

NO SUGAR ADDED
Ice cream [−sugar] + artificial sweetener =
About 180 calories per serving

ICE CREAM
Cream + milk + sugar + ingredients =
250-300 calories per serving

MENU DECODER

● **GUAR GUM AND CARRAGEENAN**

These industrial thickening agents, found in nearly every Ben & Jerry's, are used to give commercial ice cream brands their rich texture.

Häagen-Dazs

There's something amiss at Häagen-Dazs regarding their nutritional information. Their Belgian Chocolate flavour almost made it onto the Eat This section with their website stating its calorie content at just 210 per 100ml. Once we had a pot in our hands though, we saw the calorie content was actually 286 per 100ml. Häagen-Dazs say they were looking into the matter. The moral of the story? Always read the packaging.

SURVIVAL STRATEGY

The most up-to-date calorie information will be on the packaging of a product. Never trust online information fully as it can go unchecked and end up outdated.

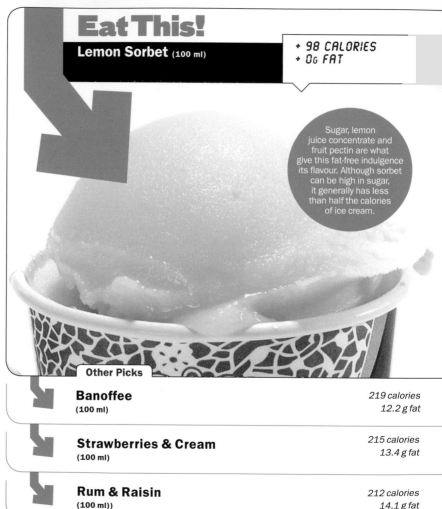

Eat This!

Lemon Sorbet (100 ml)

+ 98 CALORIES
+ 0g FAT

Sugar, lemon juice concentrate and fruit pectin are what give this fat-free indulgence its flavour. Although sorbet can be high in sugar, it generally has less than half the calories of ice cream.

Other Picks

Banoffee
(100 ml)

219 calories
12.2 g fat

Strawberries & Cream
(100 ml)

215 calories
13.4 g fat

Rum & Raisin
(100 ml))

212 calories
14.1 g fat

Not That!

Vanilla (100 ml)

+ 216 CALORIES
+ 14.7g FAT

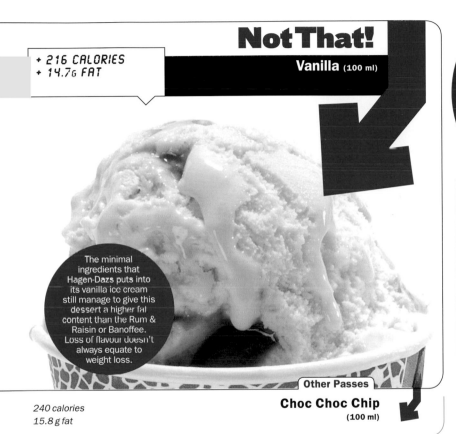

The minimal ingredients that Hagen-Dazs puts into its vanilla ice cream still manage to give this dessert a higher fat content than the Rum & Raisin or Banoffee. Loss of flavour doesn't always equate to weight loss.

Other Passes

240 calories 15.8 g fat	**Choc Choc Chip** (100 ml)
247 calories 16 g fat	**Caramel Biscuits & Cream** (100 ml)
243 calories 16 g fat	**Macadamia Nut Brittle** (100 ml)

(5)

Number of ingredients in Häagen-Dazs's vanilla ice cream.

MENU DECODER

● **SUPER PREMIUM:** Unlike Mr Whippy ice cream, Häagen-Dazs is very dense, with no added emulsifiers and comparatively little air mixed in during the production process. The product label also indicates a higher than average butterfat content.

DAZS THAT MAKE SENSE?

Häagen-Dazs is not Scandinavian, as is commonly believed. It actually originates from New York and the name is simply two made-up words designed to appear Scandinavian.

Krispy Kreme

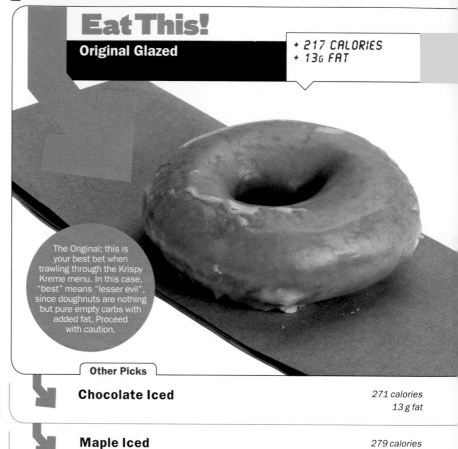

Krispy Kreme is seemingly stuck in the carb-heavy world of glazed, doughnuts. Their only other product in the UK is coffee, which you can customise with your choice of milk, cream or syrup (that's alongside a doughnut that can carry half a day's saturated fat). And don't think you can escape. Pretty soon there'll be a shop in every major town, with plans to double their UK outlets to 100 in the next five years.

SURVIVAL STRATEGY

To stay under 500 calories, you'll need to cap your sweet tooth at one filled or specialty doughnut or, worst-case scenario, two original glazed doughnuts.

Eat This!

Original Glazed

+ 217 CALORIES
+ 13G FAT

The Original; this is your best bet when trawling through the Krispy Kreme menu. In this case, "best" means "lesser evil", since doughnuts are nothing but pure empty carbs with added fat. Proceed with caution.

Other Picks

Chocolate Iced
271 calories
13 g fat

Maple Iced
279 calories
15 g fat

Apple Cinnamon
269 calories
15 g fat

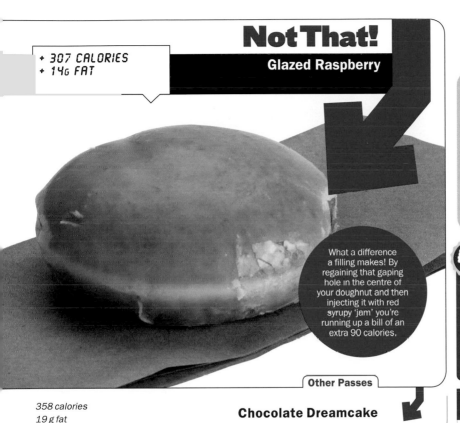

+ 307 CALORIES
+ 14G FAT

Not That!
Glazed Raspberry

WEIGHT-GAIN BOMB
The Dirty Dozen

2.604 calories
156 g fat

Ever taken a dozen doughnuts to work or home? What you have in your hands is a ticking weight gain time-bomb. Consider this; even a box of a dozen original glazed will start you out carrying a over 2,600 calorie box

What a difference a filling makes! By regaining that gaping hole in the centre of your doughnut and then injecting it with red syrupy 'jam' you're running up a bill of an extra 90 calories.

 BAD NEWS

Lost Fa(c)ts

On top of the empty carbs and added fats there is a hole, far bigger than the one in the centre of an Original Glazed—in the nutritional information. With no sat fats or sugars listed, choosing well is a bit of a shot in the dark.

Other Passes

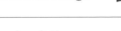

358 calories 19 g fat	**Chocolate Dreamcake**
372 calories 17 g fat	**Butterscotch Fudge**
323 calories 15 g fat	**Strawberries & Kreme**

DOUGHNUT DECODER

GLAZED CRULLER
254 calories, 16 g fat

CHOCOLATE SPRINKLES
293 calories, 13 g fat

CHOCOLATE CUSTARD
307 calories, 15 g fat

CHCOLATE KREME
339 calories, 17 g fat

121

EAT THIS NOT THAT! 2012

Chapter

4

MENU DECODER

Corner Café

WATCH YOUR ENGLISH ✘
Contains a fair whack of protein and is a good hangover cure, but everything else about this start to your day is bad. You'll take on half your recommended daily intake of fat in one go. Go veggie for protein without the fat.

THE BEST EVER OMELETTE ✔
One of the most nutritious omelettes you can eat. Feta cheese has one-third less fat than cheddar (20 grams per 100), and spinach is packed with nutrients such as vitamins A and C.

TURN PANCAKES DOWN FLAT ✘
No surprises that these sugary, buttery treats don't make a healthy breakfast. What you might not know is that a serving of sweet maple syrup also contains 10% of your salt GDA – another reason to avoid these.

GET YOUR OATS ✔
The best choice on this menu. Oats contain soluble fibre, which helps lower your cholesterol, and they're also very low in fat and sodium. Add raisins for sweetness.

BIG BREAKFASTS
Served between 7.30am and 11.30am

All our set breakfasts come with your choice of tea, coffee or small fruit juice

The Full English — £5.10
Two fried eggs, bacon, prime pork sausage, baked beans, grilled tomato, portobello mushroom and toast

The Vegetarian Breakfast — £4.95
Sauteed new potatoes, veggie sausage, two fried eggs, tomato, baked beans and buttered toast

The Lorry Driver — £6.95
Two fried eggs, two rashers of back bacon, two prime Cumberland sausages, black pudding, baked beans, mushrooms, grilled tomato, bubble and squeak, two hash browns, two buttered toast

Spinach & Feta Omelette — £3.95
Two egg omelette with feta cheese and leaf spinach

Smoked Salmon with scrambled eggs on toast — £6.95
Two eggs scrambled with smoked Scottish salmon on toast

Pancakes — £5.95
Two pancakes with red berries, maple syrup and powdered sugar

Eggs Benedict or Florentine — £5.95
Two poached eggs on an organic muffin with hollandaise and smoked ham or leaf spinach

QUICK BREAKFASTS
Served between 7.30am and 11.30am

Organic Scotch porridge — £2.50

Granola — £2.50
Honey toasted granola with Greek yoghurt & banana

Banana bread — £3.95
Warm banana bread with peaches and lavender honey

Walnut bread — £3.95
Toasted date & walnut bread with apricots and marmalade

EXPRESS LUNCH
Served between 11.30am and 4pm

Soup of the day with a buttered roll	£3.5
Home-baked ham, two eggs and chips	£5.2
Burger with fried onions and chips	£5.45
Cheese burger with fried onion and chips	£5.95
Lambs liver, bacon bubble and squeak, peas and gravy	£5.75
Steak sandwich, salad and chips	£8.45
Two sausages, mash, fried onions and gravy	£4.50
Steak & kidney pudding with chips or mash and baked beans	£4.50
Chicken & mushroom pie, chips or mash and peas	£4.50
Half a roast chicken, chips or mash and gravy	£4.95
Aged Scottish rump steak, mushrooms and chips	£12.95
Spaghetti Bolognese	£4.95
Spaghetti with plum tomato sauce and Parmesan	£4.50

Dessert

Apple pie with ice cream or custard	£2.95
Rhubarb crumble with ice cream or custard	£2.95
Chocolate pudding with chocolate sauce	£3.95
Fresh fruit salad with whipped cream	£4.50

SARNIES
served all day

On white or wholemeal brown bread. Ciabatta or French baguette 50p extra

Egg mayonnaise & onion	£2.55	Mozzarella, basil & tomato	£3.25
Cheddar cheese & onion	£2.95	Coronation chicken	£2.95
Bacon, lettuce & tomato	£3.25	Chicken & sweet corn	£2.55
Baked ham & cucumber	£3.50	Smoked salmon & cream cheese	£3.90
Tuna & sweet corn	£2.95	Prawn mayonnaise	£3.15

✖ AVOID HIDDEN MEAT
If this didn't have fatty bacon it'd be a great meal. Liver is an excellent low-fat protein source, rich in iron for healthy blood, and vitamin A to protect your eyes. Swap the bubble and squeak for mash and you've got a superfood platter.

! YOU DON'T NEED CHIPS WITH IT
If there's an option to have mash instead of chips you'll save at least 10 grams of fat per portion. Just having breakfast? A Full English isn't supposed to have chips. Lose them.

✔ PASTA BEST
Don't be fooled. Pasta dishes aren't always unhealthy. This classic is low in calories and fat as there is no cream in the sauce. And tomatoes are full of cancer-fighting antioxidant lycopene.

✖ AVOID FANCY BREAD
You'll probably get charged extra, and you'll pay with extra calories, too. Not only that, white flour has a high GI, meaning your body will absorb it quickly and turn those calories into fat.

✔ DO A NO-MAYO SANDWICH
In a greasy spoon café the sandwich range is likely to go heavy on the mayo or cheese, which means lots of extra calories and fat. If you can find, or create, one that doesn't have either, you're onto a winner.

Italian

✔ LOVE OLIVE OIL

A prime ingredient of the Mediterranean diet and rich in monounsaturated fat, olive oil is a natural juice that retains all the vitamins and healthy properties of the olives. Great for dipping or drizzled on your salad, this is the widely known secret behind the Italians' long life and healthy hearts.

✔ GET GRILLING

Grilling is one of the healthiest cooking methods, allowing those fatty juices to drain away while still retaining the full flavour of the food and serving up a much better dietary conscience. Always consider meat cooked this way.

✘ CARBONARA TAX

Abundant in saturated fats due to its heady ingredients list of bacon, cheese, butter and eggs, Cabonara can, in fact, provide your entire guideline daily amount of 20 grams of saturated fat in a single meal.

Antipasti

Garlic Bread £2.80
With Tomato, Garlic & Olive Oil

Insalata "Pierino" £6.00
Mixed Salad with Tuna Fish & Olives

Antipasto all'Italiana £6.90
Selection of Italian Hors-d'Oeuvres

Avocado con Gamberetti £5.40
Avocado with Prawns

Tonno e Fagioli £6.20
Tuna Fish, Beans & Onions

Pollo alla Griglia £6.00
Grilled Chicken topped with fresh tomatoes, basil, onion, garlic and extra virgin olive oil.

Melanzane alla Parmigiana £5.90
Aubergines with Tomato & Mozzarella Cheese

Minestrone £3.90
Vegetable Soup

Tricolore Salad £6.40
Tomato, Mozzarella, Avocado

Pasta & Risotto

Cannelloni al Forno £7.20
Pancakes filled with Meat & Vegetables

Lasagne Verde £7.20
Green Lasagne with Meat, Cheese & Tomato Sauce

Spaghetti Napoletana £7.00
With Tomato Sauce

Spaghetti al Pesto £7.20
With Pesto (Basil Sauce & Garlic)

Spaghetti alla Bolognese £6.90
Spaghetti with Meat Sauce

Spaghetti alle Vongole £7.80
Spaghetti with Clams, Garlic, Tomato & Wine Sauce

Spaghetti alla Carbonara £7.40
With Bacon, Egg, Cheese & Cream

Tagliatelle Casalinga £7.20
Egg Noodles with Ham, Mushrooms & Tomato Sauce

Rigatoni all'Amatriciana £7.20
Rigatoni with Bacon, Onions & Tomato

Rigatoni Casalinga £7.20
Rigatoni with Ham, Mushrooms, Peas & Tomato Sauce

Ravioli alla Crema £7.90
Meat Ravioli with Cream Sauce

Ravioli Napoletana £7.90
Meat Ravioli with Tomato Sauce

Ravioli alla Bolognese £7.90
Meat Ravioli with Meat Sauce

Risotto alla Piemontese £7.10
Italian Rice with Peas, Mushrooms, Peppers Tomato & Cheese

Risotto alla Marinara £8.30
Italian Rice with Seafood, Tomato & Garlic

Ricotta Gnocchi £8.30
Gnocchi with Sausage & Fennel Ragu

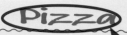

Pizza

Pizza Margherita £6.20
With Tomato & Mozzarella Cheese

Pizza Napoletana £6.20
With Tomato, Capers, Anchoives,
Oregano & Mozzarella

Pizza Pescatora £7.80
With Tomato, Prawns, Calamari
& Mussels

Pizza Quattro Stagioni £7.20
With Artichokes, Olives, Ham,
Mushrooms & Mozzarella Cheese

Pizza Nettuno £7.80
With Tomato, Tuna Fish, Onions,
Olives, Capers and Mozzarella

Pizza Quattro Formaggi £7.20
With Tomato, Bel Paese,
Gorgonzola, Parmesan & Mozzarella

Pizza al Prosciutto Cotto £7.20
With Tomato, Ham & Mozzarella

Pizza Calzone £7.50
Folded Pizza with Tomato, Ham,
Mushrooms, Egg & Mozzarella

Secundo

Scaloppa alla Milanese £10.20
Veal Escalope in Breadcrumbs,
served with Spaghetti

Piccatine Iolada £10.20
Veal Medallions with Cream,
Artichokes, Wine Sauce and Veg

Sovrana di Pollo Milanese £9.30
Breast of Chicken fried in
breadcrumbs

Sovrana di Pollo "Pierigo" £9.30
Breast of Chicken with Mushrooms,
Onions, Tomato, Garlic & Wine Sauce

Sovrana di Pollo "Claudio" £9.30
Breast of Chicken with Aubergine,
Tomato & Parmesan Cheese

Pollo alla Cacciatora £9.30
Chicken Casserole in Tomato,
Mushrooms, Onion served with Rice

Dessert

Panna Cotta £4.20
Set vanilla cream with Amarena
cherry syrup

Crepes di limoncello £5.20
Crepes with limoncello syrup and
ice cream

Tiramisu £4.90
Rich sponge, coffee liquer and
mascarpone dessert

Affogato £4.50
Vanilla ice cream served with a shot
of espresso

✓ GET TO FIRST BASE

The two extremes of the pizza base spectrum: one (marinara) has no cheese, and the other (white) has no tomato sauce. The marinara is the better choice because that red sauce is packed with vitamins and very few calories. Try it. You'll be surprised how little you miss the cheese.

! MADE TO SHARE

Worried about stocking up on calories before the main course? Share an antipasto salad with the table instead: It's loaded with high-quality protein

✗ BEWARE ITALIAN DESSERTS

All are unhealthy cream based desserts, high in calories, fat and saturates. Maybe you can pick something up on the way home instead?

✓ PARMESAN FAN

Parmesan is high in fat, so approach with caution. Nevertheless it's an excellent source of protein and calcium. It's maybe best sprinkled on top rather than included in a dish, though.

SAUCE DECODER

THE GOOD, THE BAD AND THE LARDY

Listed in ascending order of destructiveness:

Tomato Virtually fat-free, plus cooked tomatoes are a proven prostate protector.

Pesto High in fat, but most of that is healthy monounsaturated fat from olive oil. Plus basil and garlic both contain cancer-fighting compounds.

Clam The simple rule: Red is good; white is bad.

Alfredo Butter, cream, and cheese on pasta amount to 860 calories and 45 grams of fat per serving.

Mexican

✔ GUAC-ATTACK

Avocados are high in fat, but the monounsaturated kind, so they're good for your heart. They also contain vitamin E, a disease-fighting antioxidant.

✔ CHOOSE A MEAN BEAN BURRITO

Ask about the type of beans. If they're whole, this could be the healthiest thing on the menu. (The fibre in beans lowers cholesterol and helps make you feel full.) If they're refried (mashed and cooked in lard), you're better off with the chicken burrito.

✗ MOJADO NO-NO

It means "wet" in Spanish, and normally denotes a burrito that is shrouded in melted cheese and then drowned in a rich, salty tomato- and chilli-based sauce.

✔ BE A TACTICAL FAJITA EATER

A heap of onions and peppers is a plus, but skip the cheese and the sour cream – it will save you 300 calories and 15 grams of fat. To slice additional calories, ask for just one tortilla and stuff it full.

Starters

TAQUITOS (2) Corn Tortilla or
FLAUTAS (2) Flour Tortilla
Your choice of any meats, garnished with Guacamole 4.25
NACHOS 1/2 SIZE Felipe's Beans, served over a bed of Chips, topped with Melted Cheese and Guacamole   Plain 4.00   Meat 5.00
QUESO FUNDIDO [Cheese Fondue] Melted Cheese with your choice of meat, garnished with Avocado & Green Onion. Served with Tortillas.   Plain 5.75   Meat 6.75
CHIPOTLE CHICKEN WINGS (Felipe's Favorite) Wings simmered and sautéed in Alma's Chipotle Sauce. Has a Kick To It! 7.95
CABICHE COCKTAIL Fish marinated in Felipe's Homemade Cocktail Sauce & Limes. Garnished with Cilantro, Tomatoes, Onions, and Avocados. Want it Spicy? Just ask. 7.50
COCTEL DE CAMARON [Shrimp Cocktail] Shrimp prepared in its own broth, garnished with Tomatoes, Onions, Cilantro, and Avocados 8.50
ANTOJITOS PLATTER A combination of Taquitos, Flautas, Mini Tacos, Quesadillas, Chicken Wings, Tostaditas and Nachos. 10.50

Mains

All Mexican Dishes available with your choice of any of the following

CARNITAS The best carnitas in town. Pork simmered for hours with spices to create a tender succulent taste
ASADA Steak marinated with Felipe's special seasoning and grilled to order
POLLO Skinless and boneless chicken cooked and marinated with Felipe's Achiote seasonings
CHILE VERDE Diced pork cooked in tomatillo sauce
PESCADO Fish grilled with garlic butter and salsa mexicana
ENSENADA Fish lightly battered
CAMARON [shrimp]
FAJITAS CAMARON Grilled to order. A combination of roasted bell peppers, tomatoes and onions, sauteed with achiote sauce. Want it spicier? Just ask!
EN CHIPOTLE Grilled shrimp sauteed in Felipe's chipotle sauce. Very spicy.
MACHACA Sautéed strips of pork, eggs, bell peppers, tomatoes, onions and seasonings
CARNE DESHEBRADA Shredded beef simmered for hours with a touch of wine and Felipe's spices
FAJITAS ASADA Combination of strips of steak, bell peppers, tomatoes and grilled onions
FAJITAS POLLO Combination of chicken, bell peppers, tomatoes and onions grilled to order
PICADILLO Ground beef simmered with diced tomatoes and onions and lightly seasoned
VEGETARIANO A combination of grilled vegetables and lightly seasoned
CHORIZO CON PAPAS Mexican sausage grilled to order with potatoes and onions

A La Carte

TACOS
All tacos are served on a soft flour tortilla with cheese and lettuce. Hard shell or corn tortilla by request.

Taco filled with...
- Asada, Fajitas Asada 3.50
- Carne Deshebrada, Carne Deshebrada, Carnitas, Pollo, Picadillo, Fajitas Pollo, Chorizo con Papas, Nopales, Machacha, Chile Verde 3.25
- Ensenada 3.50
- Camaron 4.75

TACO SALAD
Lettuce, rice, beef, cheddar cheese, fresh salsa, guacamole, sour cream served with or without crisp shell

BURRITOS
A meal in itself that starts with a large flour tortilla and your choice of any meat, then we add rice, beans and cheese all wrapped inside.
Burrito filled with...
- Asada, Fajitas Asada, Chile Relleno 8.00
- Carne Deshebrada, Carnitas, Pollo, Picadillo, Fajitas Pollo, Vegetariano, Chorizo con Papas, Nopales, Machaca, Chile Verde 7.25
- Ensenada or Pescado 8.50
- Camaron 9.50

BURRITO MOJADO
A flour tortilla filled with your choice of meat and beans

topped with lettuce, tomato, cheese, and your choice of red or green salsa.

AMERICANO
Grilled steak or chicken, smothered with Glazed Onions and garnished with Romaine Lettuce, Tomatoes, Cheese, Sliced Avocados & Felipe's sauce, all wrapped in a Tortilla. 7.25

- Chimichanga style, Enchilada, or Ranchero Style, or any other sauce add 2.00

TOSTADAS
A crisp corn tortilla spread with beans, your choice of entree, topped with fresh lettuce, guacamole sauce and cheese.

Tostadas with...
- Asada, Fajitas Asada 8.00
- Carne Deshebrada, Carnitas, Pollo, Picadillo
- Fajitas Pollo, Vegetariano 7.25

NACHOS
First we start with a layer of beans, add a good portion of fresh chips, add more beans, your favorite meat and cover it with melted cheese and garnished with guacamole sauce.

Nachos with...
- Asada, Fajitas Asada 8.50
- Carne Deshebrada, Carnitas, Pollo, Picadillo 7.50

QUESADILLAS
Your choice of meat and melted cheese in between two flour tortillas, garnished with guacamole.

Quesadillas with...
- Asada 8.00
- Carne Deshebrada, Carnitas, Pollo, Picadillo 7.45
- Camarones (Shrimp) of your choice 10.25

TAQUITOS AND FLAUTAS
Our homemade taquitos are made with corn tortillas and our flautas are made with flour tortillas, topped with guacamole & lettuce.

ENCHILADAS
A soft corn tortilla, stuffed with cheese or meat, and smothered with enchilada sauce or tomatillo sauce then topped with melted cheese and lettuce.
Enchiladas with...
- Carne Deshebrada, Carnitas, Pollo 4.25
- Cheese 4.25
- Camaron 4.75

CHILE RELLENO
A Chile Poblano stuffed with cheese and topped with special sauce.

MOLE
Mexico's national mole dish. A blend of chillies, almonds, peanuts and filberts. Served with chicken.

✔ GO SOFT ON TACOS
Lower in fat than a hard shell tortilla. But can still pack more than 250 calories. For an even better option, ask them to make your tacos with corn tortillas; every Mexican restaurant has them to make enchiladas, and they'll cut another 100 calories from each taco.

✘ ALL SALADS ARE NOT EQUAL
It's a huge fried tortilla shell with minced beef, cheese, sour cream, and a few token shreds of iceberg lettuce. The result: 900 calories, 55 grams of fat, and perhaps the most liberal use of the word "salad" ever.

✘ DON'T GET STUFFED
Typically, enchiladas are tortillas dipped in hot fat, stuffed, rolled, covered with sauce and cheese, and baked. When topped with sour cream, two of them carry over 700 calories, 55 percent of which comes from fat.

✔ THE MOLE TRUTH
A complex sauce containing up to 40 ingredients, including chillies, ground nuts, spices, and often chocolate. Smothering grilled chicken or enchiladas, it's a vast nutritional improvement on melted cheese and sour cream.

BarFood

✓ OLIVES FOREVER

These little green wonders are a great source of antioxidant and anti-inflammatory phytonutrients and a host of other health enhancers such as phenols (tyrosol and hydroxytyrosol) and several terpenes. Although the content may change depending on your olive variety, this is your healthiest bar snack by far.

✗ BREADED MUSHROOMS

Although there is a lot to be said for the nutritional value of mushrooms, even light breading normally involves a vat full of oils and the addition of lots of salt. And then there's the mayo…

✓ GO THE CHILLI ROUTE

A good choice, since it's one of the few items in a bar that's spared the fry treatment. Ask if it's vegetarian or beef chilli, but either way you're okay. The former will be lower in fat, but the latter will be packed with protein, zinc, iron, and vitamin B12. Swapping chips for a jacket potato makes this a high-quality meal.

For Sharing

Our grazing dishes are ideal as a starter, side or perfect to share with friends

CHOOSE ANY TWO DISHES FOR £7.50 OR THREE FOR £11.50

HAND CUT POTATO SKINS
Your choice of garlic & parsley mayo or BBQ dip.

CHICKEN & CHORIZO SKEWERS
Grilled skewers with garlic & parsley mayo.

NACHOS
Topped with tomato salsa, guacamole, sour cream, jalapeños.

OLIVES & FETA
Juicy queen green and Kalamata marinated olives with roasted red peppers and feta cheese.

CAJUN CHICKEN WINGS
Spicy chicken wings with sour cream or BBQ sauce.

BREADED MUSHROOMS
With garlic & parsley mayo.

HOMEMADE FALAFELS
With yoghurt & mint dipping sauce and a squeeze of fresh lemon.

CHILLI & CHIPS
Chilli con carne and chips with sour cream

MINI SCAMPI & CHIPS
Chunky homemade tartare sauce and a wedge of lemon for squeezing.

CRISPY CALAMARI
With garlic mayo.

TEMPURA BATTERED KING PRAWNS
Freshly battered and served with sweet chilli sauce for dipping.

HOMEMADE BABY FISHCAKES
Smoked haddock, salmon, pollock, parsley & chive fishcakes with a lemon & herb dipping oil.

CRISPY JALAPEÑO PEPPERS
Stuffed with cream cheese, coated in bread crumbs. (V)

HOMEMADE FISH FINGERS
With chunky homemade tartare sauce

From the grill

OUR FRESH RANGE OF BURGERS
Homemade to a unique recipe using 100% prime beef, our burgers come with fresh tomatoes, little gem lettuce, red onion and mayo served in a floured bun with skinny fries. How proper burgers should be.

Choose either our 4oz or 8oz beef burger. Got the taste for something extra? Treat your burger to a topping or three!

BLT SANDWICH
Dry-cured bacon, tomato, little gem lettuce, red onion and mayo in your choice of toasted white or wholegrain bread.

CAJUN CHICKEN SANDWICH
Pan-fried chicken breast coated in Cajun spices, with mixed leaves and sweet chilli mayo.

SWEET CHILLI CHICKEN SALAD
Chicken breast marinated in sweet chilli sauce, with cherry tomatoes, red onion, baby spinach, radicchio and our house dressing.

CHICKEN CLUB SANDWICH
Roasted chicken, dry-cured bacon, tomato, little gem lettuce, red onion and mayo in your choice of toasted white or wholemeal bread.

✔ BUILD THE RIGHT BURGER
The difference between a hamburger with ketchup, mustard, and lettuce and a cheeseburger with mayo is 250 calories and 20 grams of fat. You can have the burger, as long as you show some restraint.

✔ BLT UP
Not as bad as you might have thought. If you pick off a slice or two of bacon and substitute mustard for the mayonnaise, you drop from 400 to 250 calories and cut the fat in half.

! SIDE ORDERS
You can make a meal out of a side order. What about a baked potato and fresh vegetables? A little hot sauce will make even that simple dish taste right for the pub.

✔ CHECK YOUR CHICKEN SALAD
This could be the best or the worst meal in the bar, depending on how it's served. If the chicken is fried and tossed with a creamy dressing, you're looking at 800 calories or more. Make sure the chicken's grilled, opt for a light vinaigrette, and you'll keep this one around 500 calories.

✔ JOIN THE RIGHT CLUB

A few key choices can redeem the club sandwich: going light on bacon and mayo, and opting for wholemeal bread makes this a winner.

Sushi

✔ MAKE MINE EDAMAME

High in protein and fibre and very low in calories, these steamed soybeans make a good start to a meal. Restaurants tend to dust them heavily in salt before sending them to your table; ask the server for your edamame salt-less, and apply it carefully yourself.

✔ BACK A YAKITORI

Skewers of lean meat and vegetables give you maximum nutrition for minimum calories. Couldn't be a better start to a meal: protein- and nutrient-packed and grilled over an open flame.

✔ CALIFORNIA DREAMING

The most popular menu item is also one of the most healthy. Just 300 calories for eight pieces, plus a dose of healthy fat from the avocado.

✘ BREAK THE HOUSE

House salad sounds healthy, doesn't it? The iceberg lettuce it's served on offers very little nutritionally, and 2 tablespoons of the oily ginger dressing can have up to 200 calories and 10 grams of fat. Instead, try some of the seaweed salad, one of nature's most potent multivitamins.

Appetizers

House Salad
Edamame
Avocado Salad
Spicy Tako Salad
Spicy Shrimp Salad
Ika Sansai
Seaweed Salad
Yakitori (chicken, beef, pork, seafood)

Roll Appetizer (3pcs California roll, 3pcs crab salad roll, 3pcs takka maki, 3pcs negi hamachi)
Sashimi Appetizer Combo (tuna, white fish & octopus)
Sushi Appetizer Combo (nigiri: tuna, white fish, shrimp, crabstick & 2 pcs tekka maki)
Sunomono (choice of: crab, octopus or shrimp)

Specialty Rolls

Black & White (white fish tempura, scallions, black sesame seeds & seaweed)
Buddy Buddy (tuna, hamachi & wasabi tobiko topped with fresh salmon & ikura)
Grand Canyon (unagi, avocado & cucumber topped with broiled white tuna, masago & silver sauce)
Green Dragon (Alaska king crab, unagi & tempura crunch with avocado)
Hawaiian (spicy salmon, tempura crunch & cucumber topped with avocado & tuna)
Jumbo (crabstick, cucumber, hamachi, unagi & masago)

Fire Island (California roll & tempura crunch topped with spicy tuna & scallions)
Fuji Volcano (shrimp tempura topped with unagi & spicy masago sauce)
Matsu (unagi, avocado, crabstick, tamago & masago)
Rainbow (California roll topped with tuna, white fish, smoked salmon, shrimp & hamachi)
Snow Mountain (shrimp tempura & cucumber topped with Alaska king crab & masago)
Tekka Tuna (spicy tuna, tempura crunch topped with tuna sashimi)

Hand Roll Special

3 hand rolls
One tuna, one yellowtail & one crab salad roll
Cooked Sushi Combo
Pieces of nigiri to include: shrimp, octopus, crab stick, tamago, smoked salmon & a crab salad roll
Chirashi
Assorted Sashimi on a bed of sushi rice
Rolls Rolls Rolls

Three pices of each: Tekka maki, negi hamachi maki, California roll, Mexican roll, Alaska roll, Philadelphiaroll and 4 pieces of futomaki
Deluxe Sashimi
3pcs blue fin, fresh salmon, hamachi, white fish, tako & 2 pcs kani & tamago
Omakase
Chef's choice of Sashimi

Don Buri

Sashimi on a bed of sushi rice served with House Salad & Miso Soup

Tekka
Ikura

Hamachi
Fresh Salmon

Sushi Combinations
Served with Miso Soup & Salad

Matsu Sushi Dinner
California roll, spicy tekka maki, 5pcs nigiri sushi consisting of: tuna, shrimp, white fish, tamago and smoked salmon

Traditional Sushi & Sashimi Dinner Traditional Sushi Dinner plus sashimi appetizer

Traditional Sushi Dinner
Nigiri sushi consisting of: tuna, white fish, mackeral, smoked salmon, yellowtail, shrimp, octopus, crab stick, tamago, crab roe & tekka maki

Nigiri & Sashimi
One serving consists of two pieces

Alaska King Crab
Amaebi (sweet shrimp)
Blue Fin Tuna
Ebi (boiled shrimp)
Escolar (seared fatty white tuna)
Hamachi (yellowtail)
Hirame (fluke)
Hotategai (scallop)
Hokkigai (surf clam)
Ika (squid)
Ikura (salmon roe)
Kanikama (crab stick)
Kanpachi (wild yellowtail)
Masago (crab roe)
Saba (Spanish mackeral)

Shake (fresh salmon)
Shake (smoked salmon)
Spicy Tuna (original or jalapeno)
Spicy scallop (original or jalapeno)
Suzuki (bass)
Tai (red snapper)
Tako (boiled octopus)
Tarako (cod roe)
Tamago (layered chicken eggs)
Tobiko (flying fish roe)
Unagi (fresh water eel)
Uni (sea urchin)
Wakame (seaweed)
Quail egg

Maki Sushi
One serving consists of 6 pieces unless noted

Alaska Roll (smoked salmon, cream cheese & masago)
California Roll (crab stick & avocado)
Crab Salad Roll
Futomaki 4 pcs (crab stick, shrimp, tamago, pickle & cucumber)
Gobo Maki (pickled burdock)
Ikura Maki (salmon roe)
Kampo Maki (oriental squash)
Kappa Maki
Mexican Roll (boiled shrimp & avocado)
Negi Hamachi Maki (yellowtail & scallions)
Natto Maki (fermented soybeans)
Philadelphia Roll (smoked salmon, cream cheese & masago)

Sake Kawa Maki (smoked salmon skin & cucumber)
Shrimp Tempura Maki 4 pcs (shrimp tempura, cucumber & crab roe)
Spicy Scallop Maki (original or jalapeno)
Spicy Tekka Maki (spicy tuna original or jalapeno)
Spider Maki 4 pcs (soft shell crab roll & masago)
Takuwan Maki (pickled radish)
Tsunamayo Maki (tuna roll)
Unagi Maki (fresh water eel)
Ume Maki 2 pcs (plum paste & oba leaf)

✔ FISH FOR COMPLIMENTS
The Japanese live longer than anyone on the planet. The reason? Fish. Nigiri is individual pieces of fish draped over rice; sashimi is just pieces of raw fish. Save yourself the unnecessary carbohydrates and go straight for the plain fish.

✗ DON'T GO TOBIKO
The Japanese word for flying fish eggs. A tablespoon of the neon-colored stuff contains approximately 20 percent of your daily cholesterol. Limit yourself to one tobiko-strewn item per sushi session.

✔ MAKE IT MACKEREL
Often overlooked in favour of more glamorous fish like salmon and tuna, the humble mackerel has twice the amount of heart-healthy, inflammation-reducing, cancer-fighting omega-3 fatty acids as salmon, making it one of the healthiest fish in the sea.

✗ PICK A DIFFERENT TUNA
This spicy roll dunks your healthy tuna in big dollops of mayonnaise. Ditch the fatty mayo and go for something just hot and fiery instead. You can even ask for extra metabolism boosting chilli sauce on the side.

Gastro Pub

STARTERS

Creamed smoked haddock soup, soft boiled quail's egg, chives £6.50

Roast butternut squash, goat's cheese croquettes, crisp shallot, pine nuts £7

Wild Yorkshire hare, mallard and partridge terrine, bilberry chutney £8.50

Herefordshire snail, bacon and creamed wild mushroom pie £9.50

Devilled Cornish sprats, tartare sauce, lemon £7.50

Grilled Scottish salmon, smoked salmonl rillette, baby gem £8

Potted Dorset brown crab and shrimps, pickles and sourdough £9.50

Oysters, red wine shallot vinegar, lemon

Dorset Rocks	*Maldon Natives*
For six £13.50	For six £14.50
For twelve £25	For twelve £27
For eighteen £36	For eighteen £38

MAINS

Beetroot tart fine, parsnip purée, roasted walnuts £13.50

Pan fried fillet of Atlantic stone bass, salt cod ravioli, watercress, tenderstem broccoli, horseradish sauce £18

Cornish fish stew £22.50

12 hour slow braised Welsh lamb shoulder, celeriac fondant, curly kale, braising juices £19.50

OIL RIGHT

It's recommended that you consume a portion of oily fish twice a week, and salmon is a great place to start. High in omega-3 acids such as eicosapentaenoic acid (EPA) and docosahexaenoic acid (DHA) it is also an abundant source of protein and amino acids, aiding muscle growth.

MINERAL CATCH

So they may not quite be the mighty aphrodisiac they are purported to be, but a small batch of 4 or 5 medium oysters will supply your daily allowance of calcium, zinc, manganese, phosphorus, iron, copper, iodine and magnesium. Phew.

CHEESE BOARD

Though cheese can provide energy, protein, calcium and a good range of vitamins from A to B (and a little B2 and 12), a board of mixed varieties can be a Russian roulette of hidden saturated fat contents that's definitely not ideal for the faint hearted.

Oxtail and kidney suet pudding with oyster a'top, mashed potato, Savoy cabbage and beef jus £21

Glazed Kilravock Farm pork, crisp pig's head, Dauphinoise potato, pickled cabbage, gravy £22.50

35 day aged Black Angus rib-eye steak, Béarnaise sauce, watercress and hand cut chips £28

Air dried rib of Longhorn beef for two people, garlic snails, Béarnaise sauce, watercress, hand cut chips £65

SIDE ORDERS *(£3.50)*

Cauliflower and macaroni cheese	Garlic mash
Roast butternut squash	Hand cut chips
Curly kale	Dauphinoise potatoes
Roasted beetroot, & goat's curd	Mixed salad

PUDDINGS *(£5.50)*

Trio of tropical fruit sorbets: papaya, mango & lyche

Apple and blackberry crumble, vanilla custard

Crème caramel, chocolate cake, fresh orange

Wild honey parfait, roasted figs, honeycomb

Selection of homemade ice creams and sorbets

Selection of British and Irish cheeses, oatcakes, fruit and nut bread, chutney (£9.50 or £18 for two to share)

✗ DON'T SUET

As the raw fat from mutton or beef, suet is something of a British tradition. Served up here in savoury form with potatoes and veg, it can stack up to a milestone 1,000 calorie meal. Watch out for it in sweet dishes as well

✗ SPUD-U-DON'T-LIKE

So how do you make potatoes unhealthy? Cover them in double cream and cheese of course. A serving of these will not only slap you with a bill for 300 calories but wallop you with your entire GDA for saturated fat as well (up to 16g).

✓ LIGHT FINISH

Not just a palate cleanser, sorbet is effectively ice cream made without dairy products. That trims off almost all the fat and calories and instead serves up a concoction of sweet syrup with fruit juice or puree, with a penalty of only 175 calories per serving.

135

Steakhouse

Starters

Smoked Scottish Salmon

Lobster Cocktail

Cromer Crabmeat Cocktail

Grilled Sea Scallops Wrapped in Bacon

Tiger Prawn Cocktail

6 Dorset Rock Oysters

Jumbo Lump Crab Cake

Potted Smoked Mackerel

Lobster Bisque

Tuna Tartare

Salads

Centre Cut Iceberg

Caesar Salad

Morton's Salad

Sliced Beefsteak Tomato, Purple Onion, Vinaigrette or Blue Cheese

Chopped Salad

Vegetables & Potatoes

Steamed Fresh Jumbo Asparagus, Sauce Hollandaise

Grilled Jumbo Asparagus, Balsamic Glaze Steamed Fresh Broccoli

Creamed Spinach

Sauteed Fresh Spinach & Mushrooms

Baked Lincolnshire Jacket Potato

Lyonnaise Potatoes

Mashed Potatoes

Beef Dripping Chips

Sauteed Wild Mushrooms

Sauteed Onions

✘ SKIP AGEING

High-end butchers and steak houses hang meat for up to 45 days to allow moisture to evaporate and to break down tough muscle fibres, enhancing tenderness and flavour. Delicious, but this meat is also very fatty and expensive.

✘ DON'T GET CRABBY

Crab, or indeed any type of fish cake, sounds like a healthy starter. But they're often loaded with potato and deep fried, so not much better than chips. If you can't resist ask for yours to be shallow fried or grilled to cut fat levels in half

✔ GO VEGGIE

Steaming vegetables is one of the very best ways to preserve their nutrients. However, covering them in sauce is one of the best ways to undo all that good. Ask for yours without. Forget creamed spinach – it can carry up to 400 calories and 20 grams of fat in a single portion. And those beef-dripping chips? They'll be busting the 500 calorie mark with ease.

✘ DO GO ON HOLLANDAISE

This is a sauce of very few ingredients, but unfortunately one of those ingredients is usually a 100 gram lump of butter. This classic French indulgence now has a healthy yogurt alternative, but this option will rarely be on the menu.

✔ GET FRUITY

Ask for raspberries if they have them. They contain 50% more disease-fighting antioxidants than strawberries. Plus you're less likely to want loads of cream with them.

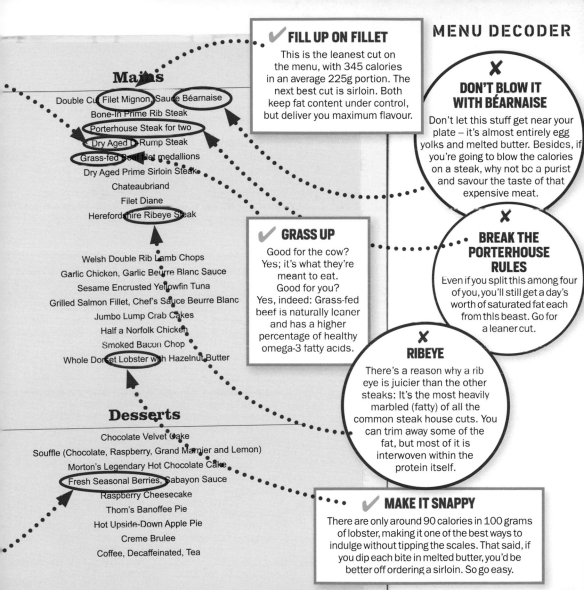

Mains

Double Cut Filet Mignon, Sauce Béarnaise
Bone-In Prime Rib Steak
Porterhouse Steak for two
Dry Aged D Rump Steak
Grass-fed Beef filet medallions
Dry Aged Prime Sirloin Steak
Chateaubriand
Filet Diane
Herefordshire Ribeye Steak

Welsh Double Rib Lamb Chops
Garlic Chicken, Garlic Beurre Blanc Sauce
Sesame Encrusted Yellowfin Tuna
Grilled Salmon Fillet, Chef's Sauce Beurre Blanc
Jumbo Lump Crab Cakes
Half a Norfolk Chicken
Smoked Bacon Chop
Whole Dorset Lobster with Hazelnut Butter

Desserts

Chocolate Velvet Cake
Souffle (Chocolate, Raspberry, Grand Marnier and Lemon)
Morton's Legendary Hot Chocolate Cake
Fresh Seasonal Berries, Sabayon Sauce
Raspberry Cheesecake
Thom's Banoffee Pie
Hot Upside-Down Apple Pie
Creme Brulee
Coffee, Decaffeinated, Tea

✔ FILL UP ON FILLET

This is the leanest cut on the menu, with 345 calories in an average 225g portion. The next best cut is sirloin. Both keep fat content under control, but deliver you maximum flavour.

✘ DON'T BLOW IT WITH BÉARNAISE

Don't let this stuff get near your plate – it's almost entirely egg yolks and melted butter. Besides, if you're going to blow the calories on a steak, why not be a purist and savour the taste of that expensive meat.

✔ GRASS UP

Good for the cow?
Yes; it's what they're meant to eat.
Good for you?
Yes, indeed: Grass-fed beef is naturally leaner and has a higher percentage of healthy omega-3 fatty acids.

✘ BREAK THE PORTERHOUSE RULES

Even if you split this among four of you, you'll still get a day's worth of saturated fat each from this beast. Go for a leaner cut.

✘ RIBEYE

There's a reason why a rib eye is juicier than the other steaks: It's the most heavily marbled (fatty) of all the common steak house cuts. You can trim away some of the fat, but most of it is interwoven within the protein itself.

✔ MAKE IT SNAPPY

There are only around 90 calories in 100 grams of lobster, making it one of the best ways to indulge without tipping the scales. That said, if you dip each bite in melted butter, you'd be better off ordering a sirloin. So go easy.

Indian

APPETISERS

Onion Bhaji	£3.50	**Samosas**	£3.25
Lamb Chops	£4.75	2 X Vegetable or Meat	
Vegetable Pakora	£3.35	**Chicken Tikka**	£3.95
Spicy vegetables deep fried with		**Lamb Tikka**	£4.25
gram flour.		Marinated and sizzling from the	
Chicken Pakora	£4.25	tandoor, served with salad and	
Diced chicken deep fried with		mint sauce.	
spices and gram flour.		**Mulagatawny Soup**	£4.95
Chicken Chaat	£3.95	A mouthwatering recipe using	
Tandoori style chicken		the finest ingredients, flavoured	
drumsticks swathed in		with sharp tamarind and tangy	
sweet 'n' sour patia sauce		tomatoes	

HOUSE SPECIALITIES

Jaipuri £7.95
A potent fusion of peppers,
onions, ginger, garlic, green
chillies and a touch of coconut
simmered in exotic jaipuri spices
Traditional Bhoona A tasty
condensed sauce with additional
ginger and garlic

Traditional Curry £7.95
Original classic on which the
ashoka Empire was born!!

Karahi Bhoona £7.95
A host of spices sautéed in a rich
tarka base with an abundance of
capsicums and onions

Malaidar £7.95
Spinach puree simmered with
lashings of green chilli and garlic,
with a dash of fresh cream.

Rogan Josh £7.95
Lamb simmered until tender in a
fusion of tomatoes, paprika and a
host of spices

Tawa Lamb Chops £7.95
Authentic lamb chops cooked
on a tawa by our master chef's
to give it a soft and succulent

flavour

Ceylonese Korma £7.95
With lashings of creamed coconut

Dum Pukht Handi £8.95
Lamb or chicken cooked in
traditional North West frontier
style using a slow and prolonged
simmering pot

Butter Chicken £8.50
Chicken breast cooked in the
clay oven then tossed in a rich
creamy, buttery, tomato gravy

Keema Matar £8.50
Authentic minced lamb cooked
with garden peas, and garnished
with fresh coriander

Saag Desi £8.50
Chicken or lamb simmered until
tender in an aromatic blend of
fresh spinach and mustard leaves

Coconut Murgh £7.95
Breast of chicken barbequed with
tandoori spices and simmered in
a rich coconut Masala

Dum Biryani £7.95
Your choice of chicken or lamb
simmered in savoury rice

✗ FALSE STARTER

These small turnovers are
stuffed with vegetables or
meat, then fried. At 200 calories
a pop for the veggie version and
more like 300 if they have
meat in, they're not an ideal
start to a meal.

✗ DON'T PICK PAKORA

Yes, they're vegetables.
But they're battered and
deep-fried before they hit
the plate, which means
they pick up a lot of excess
baggage on the way to
your mouth.

✔ SOUPS YOU, SIR

Since so many of the appetizers in
Indian cuisine revolve around potatoes
and the deep fryer, start your meal with a
bowl of soup instead. Indian soups are
broth-based and packed with vegetables,
which means plenty of nutrients and
a scarcity of calories.

✗ SLAM LAMB

Lamb is used a lot in
Indians, and most of it
comes from the shoulder or
the leg, both of which contain
a large quantity of fat. Count
on lamb mains being 200
calories more than
chicken versions.

TANDOORI DISHES

Chicken Tikka £9.95
Chicken marinated and cooked to perfection in the charcoal tandoori oven, served with rice

Tandoori Mixed Grill £13.95
A mouthwatering medley of barbequed chicken, lamb, king prawn, lamb chop served with rice and curry sauce

Seekh Kebab £10.95
Fresh minced lamb mixed with chopped onion and fresh chillies

Chicken Kebab £11.95
Chicken marinated in a hot spicy Creole-style sauce and char-grilled to perfection, served on a crisp salad dressed in mint with a curry sauce,

Tandoori Jhinga £13.95
Delicately spiced plump pacific king prawns barbecued to melt-in-the-mouth precision

Tandoori Lamb £11.95
Served with red chilli sauce and mint yoghurt

BALTI DISHES

Originating in Kashmir, these dishes are highly spiced and can be cooked medium or hot on request. Served with a Nan.

Chicken/Lamb £3.35
Chicken Tikka £3.35
Prawn £3.35

King Prawn £3.35
Lamb Chop £3.35
Keema £3.35

VEGETARIAN SPECIALITIES

Karahi Vegetables £3.35
Mixed vegetables cooked traditionally with an abundance of fresh coriander and tomatoes

Malabari Baigan £4.25
Aubergines cooked in coconut flavoured with mustard seeds

Chana Masala £3.75
Chick peas cooked with tomatoes and chef's special garam Masala

Sambar Dal £3.35
A speciality from south India, using the finest red lentils and highly flavoured with Tamarind

BREADS & RICE

Naan Bread	£2.25	Pilau Rice	£2.25
Garlic Nan	£2.95	Mushroom Rice	£2.95
Peshwari Nan	£2.95	Special Fried Rice	£2.95
Chapati	£1.95	Spiced Onions	£2.95
Tandoori Roti	£2.55	Mango Chutney	£1.15
Paratha	£2.95	Raita	£2.15
Popadom	£1.15	Seasonal Salad	£2.75

✔ CURRY FAVOUR

A great place to start on any Indian menu. Tandoori means cooked in a tandoor – a traditional clay oven that heats up to 500°C, so no oil is necessary. It's India's incendiary answer to the grill. If available, try tandoori fish or king prawns – both make for delicious meals under 500 calories.

✔ TIME FOR TIKKA

Lean chicken marinated in yoghurt and spices, this makes an excellent choice. But don't mistake chicken tikka with tikka masala. Masala means "cream" in Hindi, and that means "fat" in any language.

✔ VEGGIE DELIGHTS

Most Indian vegetable dishes are a good bet. Lentils and chickpeas add protein, and mushrooms, spinach, and tomatoes maximise nutrients. Watch out for creamy sauces, though.

✗ NAAN BETTER

The crispy charred flatbread can be more addictive than chips and salsa before a Mexican meal. Share an order with the table and have them bring it out with the meal: you'll need it to mop up the fragrant sauces.

✔ THAT'LL DAL NICELY

Find a way to make these super-flavourful stewed lentils a part of your meal – they're an excellent low-fat source of protein and fibre.

Tapas

Soups And Salads

SOPAS DEL DIA
Soups of the day – ask your server for today's choices £4

ENSALADA DE QUESOS DE CABRA
Four Goat Cheese Salad with sliced Pears, Toasted Pine Nuts, Baby Greens, and an Aged Balsamic Vinegar Reduction £5

ENSALADA DEL MONJE
Baby Spinach with imported Cabrales Blue Cheese, Toasted Pine Nuts, Red Onion, with an Aged Sherry Vinaigrette £5

ENSALADA VERDE
Seasonal Baby Greens tossed with Champagne-Citrus Vinaigrette, diced Tomatoes and Garlic-Oregano Croutons £4

ENSALADA MEDITERRÁNEA
Baby Greens, Tomato, Hearts of Palm, Sweet Bell Peppers, Avocado, Shrimp, Calamari, and Cured Bluefin Tuna Loin with White Wine Vinaigrette £6

ENSALADA DE AGUACATE Y GAMBAS
Hearts of Romaine, Carrots, Hearts of Palm, Avocado, Tomato and Shrimp with Housemade Brandy Dressing £6

Vegetables And Cheeses

ACEITUNAS Y ALMENDRAS
Assorted Marinated Olives & Marcona almonds £4

QUESO MAHÓN FRITO CON SALSA DE TOMATE
Fried Mahon Cheese with Spicy Tomato Sauce £7

QUESO IDIAZABAL CON TOMATE, ORÉGANO Y LCAPARRONES
Smoked Basque Idizabal Cheese with sliced Tomatoes, Fresh Oregano, and Caperberries £4

PIMIENTOS ASADOS EN CAZUELA CON QUESO DE CABRA
Marinated roasted Red and Yellow Bell Peppers with melted fresh Spanish Goat Cheese £5

PATATAS BRAVAS
Deep fried potatoes in a spicy sauce

BERENJENA FRITA AL SALMOREJO
Fried Eggplant with Salmorejo Sauce £6 with Serrano Ham £7

PIMIENTOS DEL PIQUILLO AL AJILLO
Sauteed strips of roasted Piquillo Peppers with toasted Garlic slivers £5

PATATAS ALI-OLI
Fried Baby Red Potatoes with an unabashed Garlic Ali-oli £4

TORTILLA ESPAÑOLA
The Classic Potato and Onion Omelette from Spain £4

✘ STOP THE CROQ
Breadcrumbs are wrapped around a filling made from a mix of flour, milk, butter, and cheese or ham, and then the whole package is deep-fried. Think: fat bomb.

✔ GO NUTS
Along with a glass of vino, almonds and olives are a traditional start to a Spanish meal. And it's a good one. All three of the beloved Spanish staples help fight off cardiovascular disease. No wonder Spaniards live longer than nearly everyone else on the planet.

✘ COSTA BRAVAS
Patatas Bravas are Cubed, fried potatoes covered with garlic mayo and hot sauce. Want heat? Go with roasted piquillo peppers instead.

✔ TORTILLA ESPAÑOLA
Ubiquitous staple of the tapas menu, this Spanish-style omelette gives paella a run for its money as the national dish. Made simply of egg, onion, and potato, it's a safe haven for confused and calorie-conscious diners alike.

Fish And Seafood

PAELLA DE MARISCOS
Prawns, mussels, squid, peppers, peas and onions served in a rich saffron rice. £6

PEZ EN ADOBO
Fresh Mahi-Mahi, cubed and marinated in the style of Cadiz, battered and perfectly fried £5

GAMBAS AL AJILLO
Sauteed Prawns with sliced Garlic and Péquin Chile Flake served sizzling hot in a Cazuela £5

CALAMARES FRITOS CON DOS SALSAS
Flash fried Baby Calamari with Spicy Tomato Sauce and Roast Garlic Caper Ali-oli £7

VIEIRAS AL VINO BLANCO CON JAMÓN SERRANO
Sautéed Scallops with White Wine and Serrano Ham £8

CROQUETAS DE JAMÓN
Serrano Croquettes with Roast Garlic-Caper Alioli and Baby Greens £5

BOQUERONES EN ESCABECHE
Fresh white Anchovy filets marinated in Garlic and Parsley £5

MEJILLONES AL VINO CON TOMATE
Steamed cultured Mediterranean Black Mussels with Herbed White Wine and Tomato Broth £5

VIEIRAS A LA GALLEGA
Baked Scallops in their own Shell with Galician Tomato, Paprika and White Wine Sauce topped with Bread Crumbs £5

Meat And Poultry

JAMÓN SERRANO
The famous mountain cured Ham of Spain. shaved to order £6

PINCHOS MORUNOS
Spicy marinated grilled Brochettes Lamb or Chicken £6

CHORIZO A LA PARRILLA CON PESTO
Grilled Chorizo Sausage with Parsley and Pine Nut Pesto £6

CHAMPINONES RELLENOS DE CHORIZO
Broiled Mushroom Caps stuffed with Chorizo Sausage and topped with Manchego Cheese £8

SPANISH MEAT & CHEESE PLATE
Chef's Selection of Spanish Cured Meats, Chorizo & Spanish Cheese £4

ALBÓNDIGAS A LA CORDOBESA
Braised Pork Meatballs in a Saffron Roast Chicken Broth £6

SOLOMILLO DE RES AL CABRALES
Grilled 3oz Filet Mignon with Blue Cheese Cream Sauce and Red Wine Carmelised Onions £7

✔ TRY PAELLA
Order the "*mariscos*" version of paella whenever possible. It's traditional along the coast of Spain and includes a clams, mussels, squid and prawns – better than the chorizo and chicken thigh variety that's also common.

✘ PRAWN AGAIN?
Prawns with a ton of garlic. A single order of these crustaceans might be sautéed in up to 60 millilitres of olive oil, which is good for your heart, but ultimately packs nearly 500 calories on its own.

✔ SHELLFISH THINKING
A good rule of thumb is to gravitate towards the shellfish. Whether steamed with white wine and herbs or served with a chunky tomato sauce, the protein fills you up while negotiating the shells slows you down. A portion won't cost you more than 400 calories.

✔ WOULD LIKE TO MEAT
A common option in Spanish restaurants. Meats are sliced super thin, so order wisely and this can be a solid beginning to a meal. Pick lean *lomo* and *jamón serrano* over fat-speckled chorizo.

Fish'n'Chips

✔ **SOUPER STARTER**

If you're lucky this will come with big chunks of protein and omega-3 rich fish (and they'll be very unlikely to be covered in batter).

✔ **GO FOR THE GRILL**

It may be the national dish, but fried fish is definitely not good for your waistline or heart. Grilled fish, in contrast, is low in fat and can lead to a 30% reduction in the risk of heart failure.

✗ **DITCH CHIPS**

Switch chips to boiled or jacket potatoes with your grilled fish and suddenly you have one of the healthiest meals around. Low in fat and high in nutrients. You need never fear an invite to the chippy again.

✗ **SQUID'S NOT IN**

Calamari to some, squid to others, should be avoided in the breaded and deep fried variety. When fried, this squishy customer contains a high amount of fat and usually a portion has 4 to 8 grams of saturated.

First Course

Soup of the day
- freshly made vegetarian soup **£3.95**

Fish soup **£ 4.95**

Crab or prawn cocktail **£ 4.95**

Deep fried camembert **£ 3.95**

Scampi **£ 4.95**

Fish cakes **£ 3.95**

Calamari **£ 4.95**

Deep fried butterfly prawns **£ 4.95**

Grilled king prawns **£ 5.95**

Melon **£ 3.95**

Taramasalata **£ 3.75**

Salmon Gravadlax **£ 5.95**

Avocado vinaigrette **£ 3.95**

Avocado crab or avocado prawn **£ 5.85**

Three course
Lunch Special
£ 9.95
(Mon-Fri)

Soup or
Prawn Cocktail

Haddock or
Cod & Chips

Ice cream

Tea or Coffee

Main Course Fish

Grilled fish on request £1.00,

All prices include chips, boiled new potatoes or jacket potato.

Fish fried in egg and matzo **£ 0.75**

Cod fillet **£ 11.75**

Haddock **£ 11.75**

Skate **£ 14.95**

Plaice **£ 11.75**

Whole plaice **£ 14.95**

Rock **£ 11.75**

Salmon **£ 11.75**

Lemon sole **£ 16.95**

Dover sole **£ 22.95**

Halibut **£ 17.95**

Rainbow trout **£ 10.50**

All fish is fried or grilled to order, please allow us time to cook it to perfection. Caution: Fish may contain bones. We use refined ground nut oil. Our food suppliers assure us that, to the best of their knowledge, none of their products contain genetically modified ingredients.

Sea bass **£ 14.95**

Calamari **£ 10.95**

Whitby Scampi **£ 10.95**

King prawns **£ 14.95**

Grilled chicken breast **£ 10.95**

Steak and kidney pie, chicken and mushroom pie or mince beef and onion pie **£ 6.95**

Half a a chicken **£ 7.95**

Battered jumbo sausage **£ 4.95**

Plain jumbo sausage **£ 4.95**

Two saveloys **£ 4.95**

Burger **£ 5.95**

Chicken burger **£ 6.45**

Side Orders

Mixed salad **£ 3.95**

Tomato and onion salad **£ 2.95**

Greek salad **£ 4.75**

Coleslaw **£ 2.25**

Mushy peas **£ 1.95**

Pickles **£ 1.95**

Homemade pea fritter **£ 1.95**

Curry sauce **£ 1.25**

Homemade Tartar sauce **£ 1.25**

Roll and butter **£ 1.95**

Heinz baked beans **£ 1.95**

Desserts

all puddings served with custard

Spotted Dick **£ 4.75**

Treacle Pudding **£ 4.75**

Chocolate Pudding **£ 4.75**

Ice cream **£ 3.95**

Home made desserts **£ 4.95**

Drinks

Tea **£ 1.25**

Cappuccino **£ 1.75**

Hot Chocolate **£ 1.95**

Fresh Orange Juice **£ 1.95**

Mineral Water **£ 1.95**

Cans – various **£ 1.15**

✗ BATTER SAUSAGE

That lovely golden crunch is unfortunately the result of soaking up a lot of fat from the cooking process. Anything deep-fried, from sausage to Mars Bars, are only making a bad thing worse.

✗ STOP AT THE SAVELOY

Sorry. You can't avoid the evils of processed meat by going for the non-battered variety. Besides the numerous seasonings and saltpeter giving it its distinctly red colour, there are about 200 calories and 17 grams of fat per sausage.

✓ MUSHY PEAS

Green is an indicator of nutritional value in veg, with peas containing vitamin K, B-1 and C. They are a rich source of dietary fibre, too.

✗ TA-TA TARTAR

Made with mayo and therefore boasts a high fat content. Complements fish but, sadly, not weight-loss.

ICE DREAM ✓

Not exactly a weight-loss food at around 300 calories a portion. But compared to high-carb, stodgy puddings, this is a good bet. Go for vanilla for the lowest calorie count of all flavours.

Chinese

APPETIZERS

A1.	Platter (for 2)	£5.25
	Egg Rolls, Chicken Fingers, Spareribs, Teriyaki Beef, Chicken Wings, Crab Rangoon	
A10.	Chicken Fingers	£5.25
A2.	Mini Pu Pu Platter	£7.95
	Teriyaki Beef (2), Boneless Spare Ribs, Chicken Wings (2), Crab Rangoon (2), Chicken Teriyaki (2)	
A11.	Boneless Spareribs	£5.25
A3.	Beef Teriyaki (6)	£5.55
A12.	Crab Rangoon (6)	£3.25
A4.	Spring Roll (2)	£2.75
A13.	Dim Sim Siu Mi (6)	£4.75
A5.	Shanghai Spring Rolls (2)	£2.95
A14.	Chicken Teriyaki	£5.55
A15.	Vegetable Spring Rolls(2)	£2.95
A7.	Chicken Wings (7)	£3.95
A8.	Fried Shrimps (6)	£5.55
A17.	Spring Onion Pancake	£2.95
A9.	Spareribs	£5.55
A18.	Prawn Crackers	£1.95

SOUP

S1.	Wonton Soup	£2.05
S5.*	Hot and Sour Soup	£2.05
S2.	Egg Drop Soup	£1.65
S6.	Chinese Vegetable Soup	£2.05
S3.	House Special Soup	£5.55

BEEF

B1.	Beef with Green Peppers	£9.55
B10.	Beef with Mushrooms	£10.25
B2.	Beef with Broccoli	£9.55
B11.*	Beef in Szechuan Sauce	£9.55
B3.	Beef with Pea Pods	£9.55
B12.*	Spicy Beef with Peanuts and Hot Peppers	£9.55
B4.	Crispy Beef with Pea Pods	£9.55
B13.*	Spicy Shredded Beef in Garlic Sauce	£9.55
B5.	Beef with Pea Pods and Bamboo Shoots	£10.25
B14.*	Hunan Spiced Beef	£9.55
B6.	Mongolian Barbecued Beef	£10.25
B15.*	Beef with Black Bean Sauce	£9.55
B7.	Beef with Scallions	£9.55
B16.*	Orange Flavored Beef	£10.55
B8.	Beef with Chinese Vegetables	£9.55
B17.*	House Special Lamb	£11.95
B9.	Sesame Beef	£10.95

* Hot & Spicy   Fortune Cookies offered by Confucius, Inc.

AUTHENTIC

Served

W1.	Moo Goo Gai Pan	£5.00
W6.*	Szechuan Spicy Bean Curd (Meatless)	£4.80
W2.*	Chicken with Vegetables in Szechuan Sauce	£5.00
W7.	Beef with Vegetables in Oyster Sauce	£4.80
W3.	Chicken with Broccoli	£4.00

PORK

P1.	Pork with Pea Pods	£5.95
P5.*	Spicy Double Cooked Pork	£6.95
P2.	Pork with Broccoli	£6.95
P6.*	Spicy Shredded Pork in Garlic Sauce	£6.95
P3.	Pork with Scallions	£6.95
P7.*	Hunan Pork	£6.95
P4.	Three Delights with Pork, Shrimp, or Chicken	£7.55

POULTRY

C1.	Chicken with Cashews	£6.05
C12.*	Strange Flavor Chicken	£6.05
C2.	Chicken with Pea Pods	£7.05
C13.*	Tender Chicken w/Black Bean Sauce	£7.05
C3.	Moo Goo Gai Pan	£7.05
C14.*	Orange Flavor Chicken	£7.75
C4.	Eight Treasure Chicken	£7.05
C15.*	Curried Chicken	£7.05
C5.	Chicken with Broccoli	£7.05

PECIALS

Served with choice of Pork Fried Rice or Steamed Rice and
n Soup. (Soup not included with Take-Out orders).

7.	Sweet and Sour Chicken, Egg Roll	£4.25
18.	Shrimp with Lobster Sauce, Egg Roll	£6.25
8.	Beef with Green Pepper, Egg Roll	£5.25
19.*	Szechuan String Beans, Egg Roll	£3.35
9.	Beef with Broccoli, Chicken Finger	£4.25
20.	Vegetarian's Delight, Egg Roll	£4.95
10.*	Spicy Double Cooked Pork, Egg Roll	£4.55
21.*	Meatless Chow Mein, Egg Roll	£4.25
	(Or choice of Chicken, Shrimp, Beef or Pork Chow Mein)	£3.55
11.	Pork with Broccoli, Egg Roll	£4.75
22.*	Shredded Beef Szechuan Style (Or choice of Chicken, Shrimp, or Pork)	£3.55

NESE LUNCH

ed Rice

W8.*	String Beans with Shredded Beef	£4.80
W4.*	Spicy Szechuan Beef With Peanuts	£4.70
W9.*	Broccoli in Garlic Sauce	£4.80
W5.*	Baby Shrimp with Peanuts	£4.70
W10.	Fried Bean Curd with Vegetables	£3.80

C16.*	Orange Chicken	£7.75
C17.*	Chef's Chicken Delight with Spicy Sesame	£7.95
C6.	Chicken with Pineapple	£8.05
C18.*	Sesame Crispy Chicken	£7.95
C7.*	Spicy Szechuan Chicken with Peanuts	£7.05
C19.*	Fresh String Beans with Chicken and Beef	£7.05
C8.*	Spicy Shredded Chicken in Garlic Sauce	£7.05
C20.*	Crispy Lemon Chicken	£7.95
C9.*	Hunan Chicken with Black Mushrooms and Broccoli	£8.05
C10.*	Chicken and Beef Hunan Style	£8.55

WEIGHT WATCHERS

All Weight-Watchers' orders are steamed. There is no
seasoning or corn starch used in cooking.

W1.	Mixed Vegetables	£4.95
W2.	Mixed Vegetables (Choice of Pork, Chicken, Beef or Shrimp)	£6.95
W3.	Broccoli or Snow Pea Pods or Asparagus	£3.95

MOO-SHI

Moo-Shi is a very popular mandarin dish which co
mushrooms, cabbage, fungus, dried lily flower, eg
meat served with 6 pancakes and Hoi Sin sa

MI.	Moo-Shi (Chicken, Beef, Pork, Shrimp, or Vegetables)	
M2.	Moo-Shi Peking Style (Spicy)	

VEGETABLES

V1.	Vegetarian's Delight	£5.55
V5.	Stir Fried Pea Pods	£5.55
V6.*	Spicy Eggplant in Garlic Sauce	£5.25
V3.	Snow Pea Pods with Water Chestnuts	£5.55
V7.*	Spicy Broccoli	£4.25
V4.	Brocoli in Oyster Sauce	£5.55
V8.*	String Beans, Szechuan Style (Meatless)	£4.25

SWEET AND SOUR

SW1.	Sweet and Sour Pork	£5.55
SW3.	Sweet and Sour Shrimp	£5.95
SW2.	Sweet and Sour Chicken	£4.55
SW4.	Sweet and Sour Combo	£7.55

DUCK

Served with pancakes, scallions and Hoi Sin sauce

D1.	Crispy Duck	
	Half	£10.00
	Whole	£17.00
D2.	Chef's Special Duck	
	Half	£10.00
	Whole	£17.00

NOODLES

L1	Chow Mein (Choice of Pork, Chicken, Beef or Shrimp)	
		£5.95
L2.	Combo Chow Mein	£5.25
L4.	Singapore Noodles	£7.25
L6.	Singapore Noodles (Meatless)	£5.95
L7.	Cold Noodles in Sesame Sauce	£5.95

RICE

R1.	Steamed Rice (White or Brown)	£0.95
R2.	Fried Rice (Choice of Pork, Chicken, Beef)	£5.95
R3.	Combo Fried Rice	£7.25

✗ DON'T GO SWEET

This cooking method means that the meat has been deep-fried and covered in a sickly-sweet pinky orange sauce. Eat with rice and it's 1,000-calories

! STICK IT TO 'EM

Always use chopsticks. They slow eating, so giving your stomach time to deliver the naturally delayed message of "I'm full, please stop" to our brains.

✓ DUCK EXTRA CALORIES

Have duck crispy and most of the fat runs out over the course of cooking, making this a healthier option than most of the stir-fry mains available. Order a side of steamed vegetables and serve it with a small scoop of brown rice.

✗ DOWN ON CHOW

Chow mein noodles are wok-fried with an abundance of oil, then speckled with fatty pork or beef. Even ordering the vegetable version won't undo the wrong wrought by this dish. Stay away.

✓ RICE GOING

Keep rice consumption to a minimum: a single portion is 300 calories. Order brown whenever possible. It will give you an extra boost of fibre and protein, which work to boost metabolism and keep you feeling full.

French Bistro

SOUPS

6 Soupe Du Jour

6 French Onion Soup

8 Soupe D'Haricot
purée of haricot verts

APPETISERS

7
Grilled Yellow Tuna Niçoise Salad
tuna, haricot verts, baby carrots, olives, pear tomatoes

5
Salade Parisienne
mixed green salad with ham, swiss cheese, artichoke hearts, cherry tomatoes and boiled eggs in a citrus herb vinaigrette dressing

6
Tomato Mozzarella Salad
fresh tomatoes, mozzarella, fresh basil, served over a small green salad with olive oil balsamic vinegar dressing

6
Roulade de Fromage de Chevre
warm goat cheese salad with potato roulade, served over a green salad with french dressing

6
Salade de Chevre Frisse
lentil bean frisee salad with goat cheese with a dusted pepper red wine shallot vinaigrette

6
Pate de Foie Gras
foie pate served over a small salad and garlic toast points

7
Escargots Au Beurre D'ail
escargots sauteed with garlic, butter, herbes and champagne

36
Fruits De Mer
Assorted shellfish with a variety of dipping sauces

ENTRÉES

13
Truit
lemon thyme roasted whole trout, spinach, shallots, in a champagne beurre blanc sauce

15
Saumon
pan seared salmon served with asparagus, carrots, julienne of vegetables, in a beurre blanc sauce

10
Lotte
sauteed monk fish in a beurre blanc sauce green pepper sauce, served with vegetables and mashed potatoes

15
Moules Provencales
steamed mussels in a white wine garlic and fresh tomato sauce, served with french fries

15
Steak Frites
grilled entrecôte steak in a classic bearnaise sauce served with small salad and chips

19
Filet Mignon
grilled filet mignon, served with baby vegetables, spinach and mashed potatoes

25
Steak Tartare
Fresh chopped beef filet served with mixed greens

21
Canard Mandarin Cerise
roasted Norfolk duck, served with sauteed garlic spinach, with cherry compote sauce

16
Confit of Wild Boar Shoulder with Mushrooms, Chestnuts And Black Currants

12
Blanc de Poulet Grand-mere
organic roasted chicken breast, served with julienne of vegetables and mashed potatoes, in a tomato sauce

14
Linguini Aux Fruits de Mer
linguini with sea food (cuttlefish, squid, octopus, shrimp, surini and mussels), fresh tomatoes, garlic and basil

13
Pappardelle pappardelle,
wild mushrooms, sage butter sweet peas, shaved pecorino romano cheese

DESSERT

5 Crêpe
with a berry sauce

5 Crème Brulée
5 Chocolate Mousse
topped with whipped cream

✔ STEAK YOUR CLAIM

Raw beef usually topped with raw egg. If you can stomach the thought, go for it: the huge protein hit goes a long way to filling you up, and because it's made with a lean cut of meat, it's relatively low in fat.

✘ BAD FIT

Popular for centuries in France, 'Confit' means the food has been immersed in fat, both to boost flavour and enhance preservation, so belt-loosening may be required.

✘ THE STEAKS ARE HIGH

A fatty cut of beef, either a rib eye or rump, topped with a pad of flavoured butter or a butter-based béarnaise sauce and flanked by a pile of fries. The damage: 1,200 calories and 70 grams of fat. Start with a steak tartare instead; it should satisfy your red meat craving for a quarter of the calories.

✘ CRÈME DE LA CRÈME

A dessert of egg yolks, heavy cream, and sugar. Lighten the load with an extra spoon, or opt for a fruit-filled crepe instead.

Thai

APPETISERS

CRISPY SPRING ROLLS (Vegetables) £5.95   FRIED WONTON (Chicken) £6.95
STEAMED DUMPLING (Chicken or vegetables) £5.95   SHU MAI (Pork & shrimp) £5.95
MEEKROB (Chicken or tofu) £7.95
VIETNAMESE SPRING ROLLS (Shrimp or tofu) £6.95   FRIED SHRIMP ROLLS £6.95
CHICKEN SATAY £7.95   PEKING DUCK ROLL £6.95

✔ HOORAY FOR SATAY

Lean grilled meat on a stick slathered in a spicy peanut sauce. Seriously satisfying, low-fat food.

SALADS

HOUSE SALAD £6.95   CHINESE SALAD £8.95
THAI CHICKEN SALAD With chicken breast topped with peanut sauce £8.95
TOFU SALAD Steamed tofu tossed with spicy lime dressing £8.95
SPICY CHICKEN SALAD Minced chicken tossed with spicy lime dressing £9.95
YUM WOON SEN Glass noodle with chicken tossed with spicy lime dressing £8.95
YUM YAI Boiled chicken, egg, and shrimp over a bed of lettuce topped with
fresh peanuts and sweet & sour sauce £9.95
SPICY BBQ BEEF SALAD Tossed with spicy lime dressing £9.95
GRILLED SHRIMP AND ASPARAGUS SALAD Tossed with house vinaigrette dressing £9.95
BBQ DUCK SALAD £9.95   SPICY DUCK SALAD Tossed with spicy lime dressing £9.95
SPICY SHRIMP SALAD Tossed with spicy lime dressing £9.95
SPICY SEAFOOD SALAD Shrimp, scallops, mussels, and crap with spicy lime dressing...£10.95

✘ NO TO TOFU

Tofu acts like a soybean sponge, sucking up anything it comes into contact with. When it's deep fried that translates into a heavy dose of oil and little else. Ask for it sautéed, or stick to vegetables.

VEGETABLES & TOFU

SAUTEED SPINACH £10.95   SZECHWAN STRING BEANS £10.95
GARLIC EGGPLANT £10.95   ORANGE TOFU £10.95
RED CURRY VEGETABLES £10.95   STEAMED VEGETABLE PLATE £10.95
VEGETABLE DELUXE Sauteed asparagus, snow peas, baby bok choy, and broccoli £10.95

✔ THAI'D TO VEGETABLES

Laced with ginger, garlic, and chilies, Thai-style vegetables pack huge flavour for few calories. Try splitting a main with a companion and sharing a side of sizzling vegetables for a great meal.

SPECIALTIES

THAI BBQ CHICKEN £10.95   BBQ PORK RIBS £10.95
ORANGE CHICKEN £11.95   TERIYAKI CHICKEN £10.95
DAVID'S SPECIAL Spicy minced chicken and fried egg on the top of coconut rice £12.95
CRYSTAL'S SPECIAL Garlic pork over chicken fried rice £12.95
PAULINA'S SPECIAL Ginger chicken and vegetables with steamed wild & brown rice £12.95
PAUL'S SPECIAL Shrimp with garlic served with asparagus and noodles £14.95
RYAN'S SPECIAL Sauteed bok choy, broccoli, and chicken with steamed brown & wild rice £12.95
MARK'S SPECIAL Stir fried flat rice noodles with scallops and eggs £12.95
FRESH ASPARAGUS & CHICKEN £12.95   MONGOLIAN BBQ BEEF £12.95
HONEY DUCK Topped with house honey and hoisin sauce £12.95
GARLIC SCALLOPS £12.95   FISH WITH BLACK BEAN SAUCE £12.95
THAI CHILLI FISH Lightly fried and topped with thai chilli sauce... £12.95
FILLET OF SOLE Lightly fried and topped with house curry sauce £12.95
STEAMED FILLET OF SOLE With house ginger and steamed vegetables £12.95
PLA LARD PRIK Crispy snapper with chili, garlic and tamarind £12.95

✘ SNAPPER DECISION

The snapper's crispy qualities come from its bath in a wok of hot, bubbling oil. Eat the whole thing with rice and the meal tops 900 calories.

MAIN COURSES

CHOICE OF CHICKEN, BEEF, SHRIMP, OR VEGETABLES £10.95

GARLIC & BLACK PEPPER Served with steamed vegetables

SPICY BASIL Served with steamed vegetables

KUNG PAO Roasted peanuts, scallion, and blacken chilli pepper

CASHEW NUT Roasted cashew nuts sautéed with scallion

BROCCOLI Sauteed with a touch of garlic

SWEET & SOUR Pineapple, onion, carrot, and bell pepper in special pungent sauce

BLACK BEAN SAUCE Our most famous sauce, bell pepper, and white onion

YELLOW CURRY (KANG KAREE) With potato, carrot, and onion

RED CURRY (PANANG) Spicy house curry sauce

GREEN CURRY Our popular curry dish from Bangkok

MIXED VEGETABLES Sauteed with a touch of garlic

PRIK KING Green beans in spicy red sauce

RICE

THAI FRIED RICE SPICY BASIL FRIED RICE

CHOICE OF CHICKEN, BEEF, TOFU, OR VEGETABLES £8.95 **CHOICE OF SHRIMP** £10.95

SPECIAL BROWN RICE Stir fried brown & wild rice with vegetables, and eggs £10.95

SEAFOOD FRIED RICE (shrimp, scallops, crab) £12.95

THE NOODLE STATION

PAD THAI Our most popular noodle dish

SPICY BASIL NOODLE Flat rice noodle with bell pepper and onion

RAD NA Flat rice noodle topped with house gravy sauce

LO MEIN Stir fried noodle with vegetables

CHOICE OF CHICKEN, BEEF, TOFU, OR VEGETABLES £9.95

CRISPY NOODLE WITH CHICKEN & VEGETABLES Topped with house ginger sauce £12.95

CRISPY NOODLE WITH SEAFOOD & VEGETABLES Topped with house ginger sauce..£14.95

BEVERAGES

THAI ICED TEA

With non- dairy creamer £2.95

THAI ICED COFFEE

With non- dairy creamer £2.95

REGULAR ICED TEA £2.95

LEMONADE £2.95

ORANGE JUICE £3.95

CRANBERRY JUICE £2.95

SODAS (COKE, SPRITE, DIET COKE) £2.95

SPARKLING WATER £3.00

BOTTLE WATER £5.00

BEERS

DOMESTIC BEER £3.25

IMPORTED BEER £3.75

HOT SAKE £3.75 **HOT TEA** £1.50

WINES

GLASS £5.95

BOTTLE £22.00

WHITE WINE CHARDONNAY, SAUVIGNON
BLANC, PINOT GRIGIO

RED WINE MERLOT, CARBERNET

PLUM WINE

✔ GREEN PARTY

Thai curries, regardless of colour, are based on coconut milk. While high in saturated fat, most of that comes from lauric acid, which has been shown in more than 60 studies to decrease your risk of cardiovascular disease. Pick a lean protein like prawns or chicken, and this makes for a healthier option than many of the noodle-based dishes

✖ DON'T BE A FRIED

Nearly as oil-soaked as its Chinese counterpart.

✔ YOUR PAD

An average portion of this popular noodle dish can pack 600 calories, but it's usually very low in saturated fat, making it a good option.

✖ PUT TEA ON ICE

Any potential benefits of this brute-strength black tea are hopelessly diluted by the addition of sweetened condensed milk and a few fistfuls of sugar. Sip this and your blood sugar levels will soar, which signals your body to start storing fat.

Chapter

5

AT THE SUPERMARKET

**EAT
THIS
NOT
THAT!
2012**

Quantum physics.

Middle East politics. The Eurozone crisis.

What do these three things have in common? Each of them is easier to understand than the average British supermarket.

No matter how meticulously edited our shopping lists are, it's hard not to be overwhelmed the minute we set foot into the electric blue fluorescent glow of our local food shop. More than 50,000 packaged goods line the shelves of the average supermarket, and that's before you take into account the meat, fish, deli, and cheese counters; the fruit and veg section, with its exotic greens and 30 different kinds of apples; the pre-cooked 'takeaway' area, where you can get a curry or a roast chicken; and the assistant with the latex gloves offering a taste of chorizo and bourbon mustard or whatever else they're pushing that day. Go in with a plan to buy 35 items, and the chances are that you'll come out with 50—and wonder the next day how they ever crept into your kitchen.

And the power of supermarkets to have their way with us has never been greater. A recent survey by Oxford University found the economic downturn means more families are eating at home, with 48 percent of us saying we eat out less frequently to save money. But are we saving? Food manufacturers are excellent at getting us to buy their products. That's why it's important for your wallet—and the part of your body that sits on it—to be smart about supermarket strategies.

Nobody wants to have to exercise discipline every time they go shopping, especially when it comes to the visceral happiness that food can bring. Yet bad judgment at the supermarket can have consequences that last a lifetime. Because we're creatures of habit, we tend to grab the same brands every time we shop. That's fine, as long as we've chosen wisely. But the wrong choices can cost us thousands of calories every year.

Consider this: Let's say that every night you have a modest dessert of a Snickers Ice Cream. That means every night you're taking in 178 calories for dessert. Not a terrible nutritional crime—more like a misdemeanour. But if your regular choice was Mars Ice Cream instead of the Snickers, and you ate it every night, by the end of a year you would have saved yourself more than 12,500 calories—the equivalent to nearly four pounds of fat.

Amazing, right? But every single choice you make in the supermarket comes with the same potential long-term consequences. Think of all the things you and your family consume on a regular basis—staples like bread, crisps, cheese, salad dressings, and ice cream. Each choice can add an unnecessary 10, 50, 100 calories or more to your day—and that can very quickly add up. (Imagine those calories were money. You'd want to know if you were spending £100 extra every day on something you didn't have to, right?)

So in this chapter, we've surveyed the supermarket shelves and found calorie savings here, there, and everywhere. For the most part we've steered clear of products branded 'light' or 'diet' as you can usually work out for yourself that these are better for weight loss. We've only included them if they are amazingly good (or, in fact, bad). Some of the other savings are little; some are dramatic, however, and you will be shocked by how quickly and easily they will change your life. So, use this chapter to rewrite your shopping list—and try some of the six simple strategies below to help you stick to it.

STRATEGY #1

STAY AWAY FROM THE SOFT, CREAMY CENTRE That would be the soft, creamy centre of the supermarket—aisles three to 11 in most shops. While the healthy stuff like dairy, fruit and veg, meat, and seafood is usually located around the edges, the interior is almost always packed with highly processed foods made with corn and soy and the 3,000 or more additives manufacturers use to make things that are edible but aren't actually food.

STRATEGY #2

AVERT YOUR EYES! On any grocery shelf, the most highly processed, most calorific, and often most highly priced products are about five feet off the ground. Why? Because that's about where your eyes are. That's very valuable real estate, and since supermarkets charge manufacturers for that placement, you can bet that the food companies are figuring out a way to pass that cost on to you—either by trimming nutrition or ramping up cost, or both. Reach up and kneel down, and you'll find both price points and nutrition labels that make a lot more sense.

STRATEGY #3

GET BACK TO THE EARTH On one hand, we have an apple, a chicken, and a potato. On the other hand, a jar of apple sauce, a bag of chicken nuggets, and some chips. Which hand is healthier?

It's pretty simple. The apple has more nutrients than the sauce, the chicken has fewer carbohydrates than the nuggets, and the potato has less fat than the chips. And the apple/chicken/potato hand is a lot cheaper, too. It's a simple rule: The closer food is to its natural form, the healthier it is for you. So until they start growing apples inside little plastic containers, stick with what Mother Nature gave you.

STRATEGY #4

EAT MORE FOOD, EAT FEWER INGREDIENTS Another important thing to keep in mind: the fewer ingredients, the better something typically is for you. (Foods with five or fewer deserve a special place in your larder.) When apples turn into apple sauce, they can often double their calories because of the addition of extra sugar. Which would you rather eat: an apple; or a combination of apples, water and sugar for twice the calories?

STRATEGY #5

WATCH THE BATTING ORDER Reading an ingredients label is like reading the cricket scores: it has plenty of information, but you need to understand what the stats mean. If you know what LBW and BF mean, you have a good understanding of what's happening in the game. If not, the statistics just read like gibberish.

Nutrition labels are the same. There are two things to keep an eye on: The first is the order of ingredients—labels by law must list them in order of volume. So if the number one ingredient is, say, "spinach," that's good. If it's "sugar" or "glucose-fructose syrup" or "canary droppings," that's probably bad. The second thing to look at is the servings per container. You'd be amazed by how a 200-calorie meal really becomes a 400-calorie meal when the little tiny dish supposedly contains two servings—even though you know you're going to eat the whole thing.

STRATEGY #6

ELIMINATE THE DAILY SHOP A recent study found that shoppers who made "quick trips" to the shops end up spending 54 percent more on groceries than they had planned. Instead, be smart about your trips. Bring a list—and a pen to cross off what you've already dropped into your trolley. And try doing your shopping on Wednesday evening—that's when supermarkets are at their quietest. This means a shorter trip and less time in the checkout aisle, eyeing the latest celebrity gossip magazines and those enticing little chocolate-covered crispy crackers that you don't mean to buy, but the children are complaining and you're hungry and...

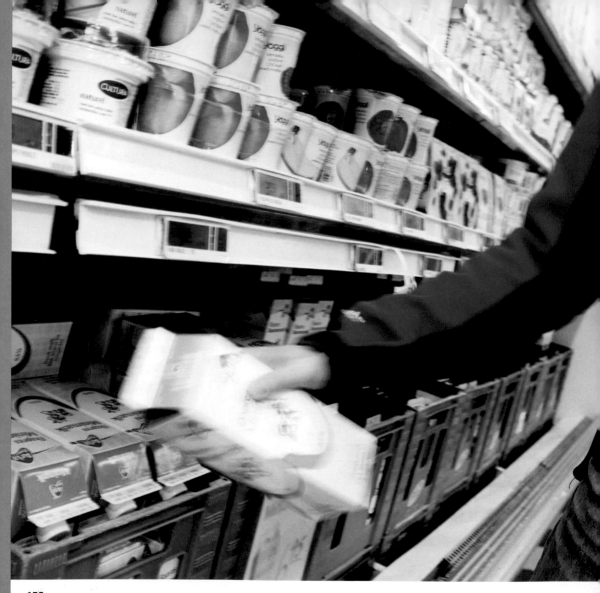

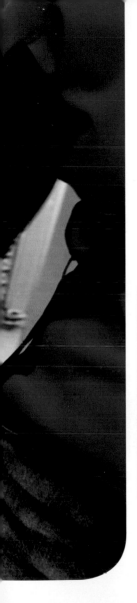

Essentials

Everyday items like bread and cereal can hide
surprisingly big calorie hits. Use this guide to
avoid them on your next trip to the supermarket

HOW TO USE THESE PAGES

Look out for our star picks on each page. The
comparison may astound or befuddle you. Who
knew two similar products could be so different?

Eat This!

Not That!

Tesco Simply Pepperoni
(1/4 pizza)
400 calories
19.3g fat
(9g saturated)
2.3g salt

Though this tasty cheese laden feast should only really be an occasional indulgence, the meaty juice item makes a surprisingly calorie-light...

The clue is in the title, this meat comes in at four different cheeses and a whopping 22g of fat.

Tesco Cheese Feast
(1/2 pizza)
650 calories
32g fat
(18g saturated)
2.7g salt

Chicago Town Miami Meaty
(1/4 pizza)
371 calories
15.7g fat
(7.6g saturated)
1.7g salt

While deep-pan can spell disaster, just a quarter of this hefty pizza should be enough to curb your cravings.

Goodfella's Stonebaked Thin Margherita
(1/4 pizza)
(9.5g fat)
(5.2g saturated)
2.9g salt

Turning to thin just to be fair stuffed variety means fewer carbs, calories and fat grams.

Waitrose Thin and Crispy Ham & Pineapple
(1/2 pizza)
440 calories
16.1g fat
(6g saturated)
1.3g salt

Opting for thin crust over the stuffed variety means lower carbs.

Ristorante Pizza Funghi
(1 pizza)
427 calories
23.4g fat
(5.8g saturated)
2.27g salt

Opting for thin crust over the stuffed variety means lower carbs, calories and fat grams.

Ristorante Pizza Pollo
(1/2 pizza)
378 calories
14.1g fat
(5.3g saturated)
2.88g salt

Opting for thin crust over the stuffed variety means lower carbs, calories and fat grams.

Waitrose Thin and Crispy Caramelised Onion & Feta Cheese
(1/2 pizza)
396 calories
20.6g fat
(16.1g saturated)
1.6g salt

Opting for thin crust over the stuffed variety.

Goodfella's Meal Feast
(1/4 pizza)
351 calories
16.4g fat
(6.4g saturated)
1.4g salt

A top of lots etc. Breaking policies really "thick" in the crust.

Chicago Town Take Away Pepperoni
(1/4 pizza)
446 calories
19g fat
(9g saturated)
3g salt

This heavyweight comes with a massive 76g fat in total. Try working that off.

Each page is constructed as a mirror image of the one
opposite. Compare similar products on each side by
reading the same coloured boxes on both pages.

Bread

Eat This!

Warburtons Wholemeal
(1 slice, 24 g)

58 calories
0.6 g fat
0.7 g sugar
1.5 g fibre

An excellent wholemeal loaf that's high in fibre, but sliced a bit thinner, so you don't end up with a plateful of unnecessary calories. The slice is right.

Warburtons Crumpets
(1 crumpet, 55 g)

98 calories
0.4 g fat
1.1 g sugar
1.3 g fibre

A crumpet outstrips a muffin by a massive 40 calories and it's only 9 grams lighter. Just don't drown it in butter.

Tesco Stay Fresh White, Medium
(1 slice, 38 g)

85 calories
3 g fat
1 g sugar
1.9 g fibre

If you're must have white, go for this decent slice. It's processed though, so even though its low in calories, your body will absorb them quickly.

Tesco Wholemeal, Medium
(1 slice, 38 g)

80 calories
0.8 g fat
1.4 g sugar
2.4 g fibre

Basic bread is where it's at when it comes to watching your weight. This has chunkier slices and a high fibre content that means slow absorption.

Hovis Original Wholemeal
(1 slice, 25 g)

56 calories
0.5 g fat
0.8 g sugar
1.3 g fibre

This is probably the healthiest slice here, however it's also the smallest, so you have to be careful that you don't just end up reaching for extra.

Marks & Spencer Super Seeded Rolls
(1 roll)

185 calories
4.3 g fat
2.1 g sugar
5.8 g fibre

These M&S rolls pack in an amazing amount of fibre, while still managing to beat the white variety on calories. They earn their super name.

Warburtons Seeded Batch

(1 slice, 46 g)

137 calories
4.1 g fat
1.5 g sugar
2.7 g fibre

All those seeds do a good job of bumping up the calories and fat, so you get a denser slice whichever way you cut it. Fibre is OK. But gram for gram standard wholemeal wins.

Not That!

Warburton Muffins

(1 muffin, 64 g)

138 calories
1 g fat
1.3 g sugar
1.8 fibre

The denser muffin loses out to its lighter crumpet cousin. The extra fat and calories make this an obvious pass.

Marks & Spencer Soft White Seeded Rolls

(1 roll)

220 calories
4.3 g fat
4.6 g sugar
2.1 g fibre

These white rolls are slightly larger than their Super Seeded rivals, but there's no extra fibre for your extra calories.

Hovis Seeded Sensations

(1 slice, 44 g)

122 calories
2.9 g fat
1.7 g sugar
2.3 g fibre

These slices are bigger than wholemeal Hovis loaf, but gram for gram you're still looking at a 20% increase in calorie load. Not a weight-loss loaf

Tesco Multigrain Farmhouse Batch

(1 slice, 50g)

130 calories
4.3 g fat
1.9 g sugar
3.4 g fibre

Another bigger slice, but also more calories per gram. Plus if your slices are bigger portion control is harder. A decent whack of fibre here, though.

Tesco White Farmhouse Batch

(1 slice, 50 g)

120 calories
0.6 g fat
1.8 g sugar
1.3 g fibre

Not too many saving graces for this loaf. Big chunky slices that are high in calories and low in fibre, so your body will turn them to fat in no time.

Cereal

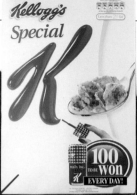

Eat This!

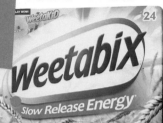

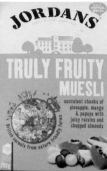

Weetabix
(2 biscuits)

134 calories
0.8 g fat
(0.2 saturated)
1.7 g sugar
3.8 g fibre

Beats newcomer Oatibix on calories and fat. Weetabix even have more fibre, which will help to slow absorption of calories.

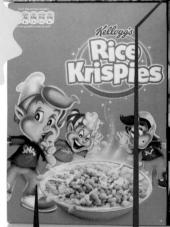

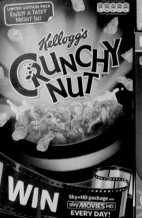

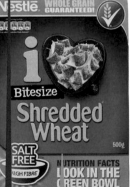

Rice Krispies
(1 bowl, 30 g)

115 calories
0.3 g fat
(0.1 g saturated)
3 g sugar
0.3 g fibre

A light morning bite that's surprisingly low in sugar. Little in the way of fibre, though.

Special K
(1 bowl, 30 g)

114 calories
0.5 g fat
(0.2 g saturated)
5 g sugar
0.8 g fibre

The weight-loss favourite is true to its marketing. But, low fibre content means there are better breakfasts.

Crunchy Nut Cornflakes
(1 bowl, 30 g)

121 calories
1.5 g fat
(0.3 g saturated)
11 g sugar
0.8 g fibre

If you want a honey treat this is the one. Packed with sugar, though.

Jordans Truly Fruity Muesli
(1 bowl, 40 g)

134 calories
1 g fat
(0.2 g saturated)
12.4 g sugar
2.6 g fibre

Fruit makes the sugar high. But calories are still under control.

Shredded Wheat Bitesize
(1 bowl, 40 g)

138 calories
0.9 g fat
(0.2 g saturated)
0.3 g sugar
4.7 g fibre

Low in fat *and* sugar *and* high in fibre. One of the best.

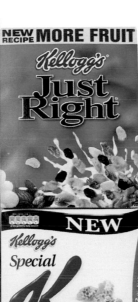

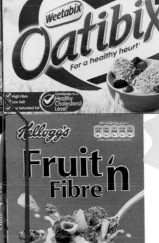

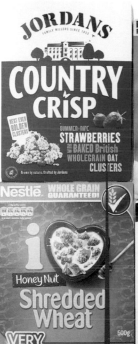

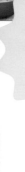

Not That!

Oatibix
(2 biscuits)

189 calories
3.8 g fat
(0.6 saturated)
1.5 g sugar
3.5 g fibre

A healthy start to your day – but original Weetabix has significantly fewer calories, so for weight-loss skip these oats.

NUTRITIONAL VALUES DO NOT INCLUDE MILK

Honey Nut Shredded Wheat
(1 bowl, 40 g)

159 calories
2.6 g fat
(0.9 saturated)
6.5 g sugar
3.8 g fibre

No surprises on the honey-nut front here.

Jordan's Country Crisp
(1 bowl, 40 g)

176 calories
3.8 g fat
(1.4 g saturated)
6.5 g sugar
2.5 g fibre

Low in sugar for a sweet one, but tips the scales with fat content.

Special K Honey Clusters
(1 bowl, 45 g)

175 calories
1.5 g fat
(0.3 g saturated)
11 g sugar
1.5 g fibre

Not-so-special thanks to honey invaders.

Just Right
(1 bowl, 40 g)

207 calories
3 g fat
(1.5 g saturated)
15 g sugar
2 g fibre

Just right for weight gain, perhaps. More calories than a Flake and nearly as much sugar.

Fruit 'n Fibre
(1 bowl, 40 g)

152 calories
2.5 g fat
(1.5 g saturated)
10 g sugar
3.5 g fibre

There's a bit of fibre, but lots of fruit pushes up the calories and sugar making this a poor weight-loss option.

Cheese

Eat This!

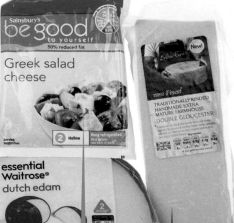

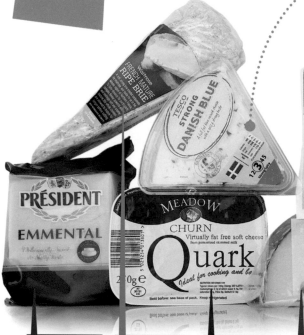

Tesco Danish Blue
(100 g)
345 calories
28.6 g fat
(18.2 g saturated)
3.8 g salt

The soft Continental blue cheese beats Stilton in calories and fat. It is salty though, so go easy.

President Emmental
(100 g)
360 calories
28 g fat

As a general rule, the softer the cheese the fewer calories. So Emmental is better than Cheddar.

Waitrose French Mature Ripe Brie
(100 g)
292 calories
22.7 g fat
(16.7 g saturated)
1.42 g salt

The most flavour for your calories. Still, take care.

Meadow Churn Quark
(100 g)
73 calories
0.2 g fat
(0.1 g saturated)
0.1 g salt

A cheesy super food! Low in everything except protein (13 grams per 100)

Waitrose Essential Dutch Edam
(100 g)
317 calories
23.8 g fat
(16.1 g saturated)
2.55 g salt

The Dutch do it better than us when it comes to rubbery cheese.

Sainsbury's Be Good To Yourself Greek Salad Cheese (100 g)
172 calories
11.5 g fat
(10.3 g saturated)
1.8 g salt

Regular feta is good, this is even better.

Tesco Finest Double Gloucester
(100 g)
395 calories
33 g fat
(20.8 g saturated)
1.5 g salt

For hard cheese it's OK. Better than Manchego, but limit intake.

162

Not That!

Tesco Blue Stilton
(100 g)
410 calories
35 g fat
(23 g saturated)
2 g salt

You can get your blue cheese fix by sidestepping this British classic and going Danish.

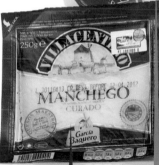
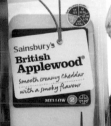
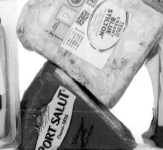
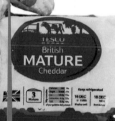

Villacenteno Manchego
(100 g)
455 calories
38 g fat
(26.2 g saturated)
0.84 g salt

A hard Spanish customer. A full 60 calories more than Double Gloucester.

Sainsbury's Italian Hard Cheese
(100 g)
408 calories
32 g fat
(24.9 g saturated)
2.06 g salt

Grate this on your salad sparingly. Or, even better, switch to feta.

Sainsbury's British Applewood Cheese
(100 g)
416 calories
34.9 g fat
(2.7 g saturated)
1.75 g salt

More flavour than Edam—but a lot more calories.

Port Salut
(100 g)
331 calories
27 g fat

This actually isn't bad (for a cheese). But compare it directly with Quark, opposite, and you can see why it falls down for weight loss.

Tesco Cambozola Blue Brie
(100 g)
426 calories
41.1 g fat
(27 g saturated)
1.7 g salt

Remarkably bad for a soft cheese. This has the most fat out of any here.

Tesco Mature Cheddar
(100 g)
420 calories
34.9 g fat
(21.7 g saturated)
1.8 g salt

A store cupboard classic. Switch this for Emmental and lose a pound of fat a year.

Cooked meat

Eat This!

Chorizo is a notoriously calorific meat, but opt for this cooks' ingredients version to minimise the damage.

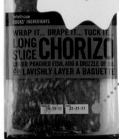

Waitrose Long Slice Chorizo
(100g)
330 calories
26.2 g fat
(10 g saturated)
4.3 g salt

Red Lion Ham
(100 g)
99 calories
2.1 g fat
(0.7 g saturated)
2 g salt

Basic slices have a lower calorie and fat count. Save money and lose weight.

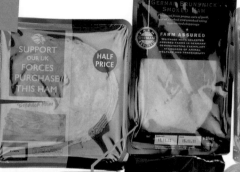

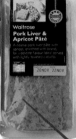

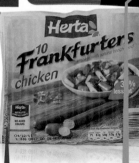

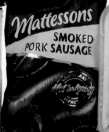

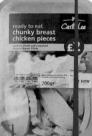

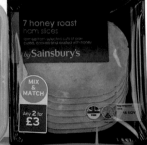

Herta Chicken Frankfurter
(1 sausage, 35 g)
71 calories
5.6 g fat
(1.7 g saturated)
0.7 g salt

One of the lowest calorie ways you can eat a sausage

Waitrose German Brunswick Smoked
(100g)
157 calories
7.8 g fat
(3.2 g saturated)
2 g salt

Half the calories and fat of salami. A meaty winner.

Matteson Smoked Pork Sausage, Hot and Spicy
(100 g)
245 calories
19 g fat
(8.6 g saturated)
2.3 g salt

Not great. But hot and spicy version cuts the calories.

Castle Lea Chunky Breast Chicken
(½ pack 100 g)
105 calories
1.3 g fat
(0.4 g saturated)
0.98 g salt

Good, honest, un-mucked-about-with chicken.

Waitrose Pork & Apricot Pate
(¼ pack, 42.5 g)
122 calories
9.65 g fat
(3.4 g saturated)
0.77 g salt

Courser pate with added fruit means less room for meat, so less fat.

Sainsbury's Honey Roast
(1 slice)
19 calories
0.4 g fat
(0.1 g saturated)
0.34 g salt

A basic slice of ham will beat a luxury version on calories, even if it's honey roasted.

164

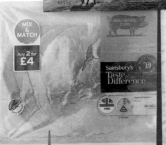

Waitrose Chorizo Ibérico
(100g)
418 calories
31.5 g fat
(11.5 g saturated)
8.5 g salt

As is so often the case, luxury branding means more calories and fat. The real surprise here is the huge hit of salt.

Not That!

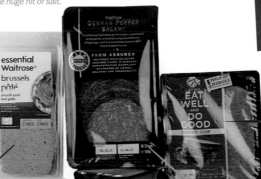

Red Lion Corned Beef
(100 g)
228 calories
14 g fat
(6 g saturated)
2.3 g salt

Seven times the fat of ham. Just hope your gran's not making sandwiches…

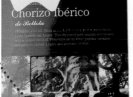

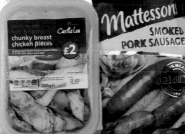

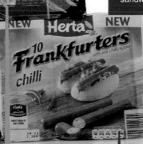

Sainsbury's Wiltshire Cure	**Waitrose Brussels Pate**	**Castle Lea Spicy Chicken**	**Matteson Pork Sausage**	**Waitrose Salami**	**Herta Chilli Frankfurter**
(1 slice)	(¼ pack, 42.5 g)	(½ pack 100 g)	(100 g)	(100g)	(1 sausage, 35 g)
40 calories	156 calories	146 calories	320 calories	333 calories	100 calories
1.3 g fat	14.9 g fat	1.6 g fat	30 g fat	26 g fat	8.8 g fat
(0.4 g saturated)	(5.4 g saturated)	(0.5 g saturated)	(11 g saturated)	(10 g saturated)	(3.4 g saturated)
0.83 g salt	0.71 g salt	1.63 g salt	2.3 g salt	4 g salt	0.53 g salt
Thicker slices, yes, but also more fat per gram. Go basic instead.	Smooth pate won't be doing your waistline any favours.	You get 27 per cent of your guideline daily amount of salt in half a pack.	Eat the whole sausage and you'll exceed your guideline sat fat in one sitting.	Salami is packed with fat. You can see it. Stick to just a slice or two to save your bacon.	Spice up your meal, and your saturated fat, with this frankfurter.

165

Cooking Sauces

Eat This!

You might think Chicken Tonight sauces are all the same. Not so. This saves nearly 100 calories over Honey & Mustard.

Chicken Tonight Spanish
(¼ jar)

56 calories
2 g fat
(trace saturate)
1.1 g salt
8 g sugar

Bisto Cheese Sauce Granules
(1 serving)

41 calories
2 g fat
(2 g saturated)
0.7 g salt
1 g sugar

Granules give more control over fat content. This can be made with water.

Coleman's White Sauce
(1 serving, with semi-skimmed milk)

63 calories
2 g fat
(1 g saturated)
0.6 g salt
4 g sugar

The lowest calorie way to make white sauce.

Blue Dragon Thai Green Cooking Sauce
(100 g)

100 calories
6.2 g fat
(4.1 g saturated)
0.92 g salt
4.9 g sugar

Creamy, yes. But fat and sugar dials are set mercifully low.

Patak's Rogan Josh
(⅓ jar, 166 g)

106 calories
5.6 g fat
(0.3 g saturated)
1.2 g salt
7.3 g sugar

Tomato-based Rogan Josh is curry king, in a restaurant—or cooking at home.

Tesco Finest Sweet & Sour
(½ jar, 180 g)

163 calories
0.2 g fat
(0.2 g saturated)
0.2 g salt
30.1 g sugar

Sweet and sour can't help but go overboard on sugar. At least this keeps fat levels down.

Loyd Grossman Bolognese Sauce
(100 g)

55 calories
2.5 g fat
(0.3 g saturated)
0.4 g salt
5.2 g sugar

You're bound to have at least 200 g so double up savings.

166

Feel like Chicken Tonight? Fine, just make sure it's not this one: it has more sugar per portion than an Aero Chocolate Mousse.

Not That!

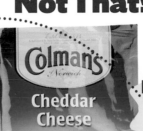

Chicken Tonight Honey & Mustard
(¼ jar)

144 calories
7 g fat
(1 g saturated)
1.6 g salt
14 g sugar

Coleman's Cheddar Cheese
(1, serving, with semi-skimmed milk)

77 calories
3 g fat
(2 g saturated)
0.8 g salt
5 g sugar

Milk helps to bump up calories.

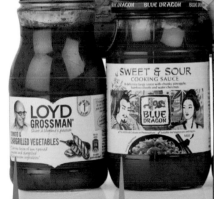

Loyd Grossman Chargrilled Vegetables
(100 g)

65 calories
3.2 g fat
(0.4 g saturated)
1 g salt
6 g sugar

A whole gram of salt in less than a portion. Best avoided.

Blue Dragon Sweet & Sour
(½ jar, 212 g)

227 calories
2.1 g fat
(0.2 g saturated)
1.2 g salt
42.8 g sugar

Nearly half your daily sugar intake in your main course. You can rule out pudding.

Tesco Tikka Masala
(½ jar, 166g)

205 calories
14 g fat
(8.9 g saturated)
0.8 g salt
11.9 g sugar

Chicken Tikka is a weight-loss hero, but masala sauce undoes all its good work.

Tesco Finest Thai Green Curry
(100 g)

140 calories
12.5 g fat
(5.8 g saturated)
1.5 g salt
1.7 g sugar

Twice the fat of its Blue Dragon rival and calories to show for it.

Tesco White Lasagne Sauce
(1 serving)

115 calories
9 g fat
(3 g saturated)
0.7 g salt
trace sugar

Twice the calories and over four-times the fat of the Coleman's mix-yourself version.

167

Crackers

Eat This!

Tuc Original
(1 cracker)
25 calories
1.4 g fat
(0.7 g saturated)
0.1 g salt

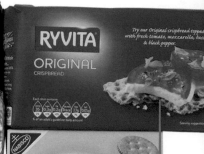

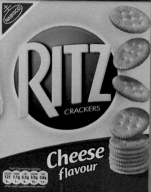

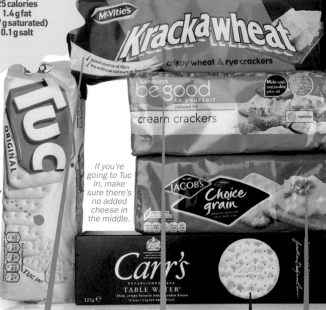

If you're going to Tuc in, make sure there's no added cheese in the middle.

McVities Krack a wheat
(1 cracker)

33 calories
1.4 g fat
(0.7 g saturated)
0.25 g salt

These add extra flavour, without the calorie jump you'll get from sweeter rivals.

Sainsbury's Be Good To Yourself Cream Crackers
(2 crackers)

32 calories
0.5 g fat
(0.2 g saturated)
0.11 g salt

You'd be crackers not to…

Carr's Table Water
(3 crackers)

42 calories
0.9 g fat
(0.3 g saturated)
trace salt

The supermodel of the cracker world: thin, classy and keeps calories under control.

Jacob's Choice Grain
(1 cracker)

32 calories
1.1 g fat
(0.5 g saturated)
0.25 g salt

A classic accompaniment to cheese. Beats fancy, flavoured upstarts.

Ritz
(25 g)

121 calories
6.2 g fat
(3 g saturated)
0.9 g salt

Pretty unhealthy these, but sneak into the Eat This side on comparison with McVities Cheddars.

Ryvita Original
(1 slice)

35 calories
0.2 g fat
(trace saturate)
0.05 g salt

A store cupboard staple since you were young and with good reason.

Not That!

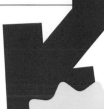

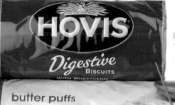

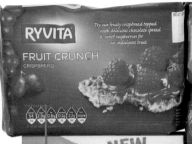

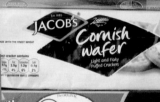

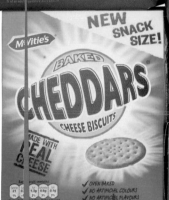

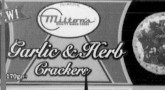

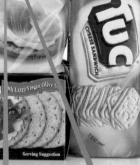

Tuc Sandwiches put cheese in the middle for you (along with 2 grams of sat fat) Wouldn't you prefer to pick your own topping?

Tuc Cheese Sandwich
(1 cracker)
72 calories
4.3 g fat
(2.1 saturated)
0.25 g salt

Ryvita Fruit Crunch	**McVities Baked Cheddars**	**Jacob's Cornish Wafer**	**Milton's Garlic & Herb**	**Sainsbury's Butter Puffs**	**Hovis Digestive Biscuits**
(1 slice)	(25 g)	(1 cracker)	(3 crackers)	(2 crackers)	(1 cracker)
54 calories	132 calories	45 calories	71 calories	50 calories	37 calories
0.8 g fat	7.9 g fat	2.7 g fat	3 g fat	2.5 g fat	2.1 g fat
(0.1 g saturated)	(5.2 g saturated)	(1.25 g saturated)	(0 saturated)	(1.2 g saturated)	(1 g saturated)
trace salt	1.5 g salt	0.25 g salt	0.3 g salt	0.1 g salt	1 g salt
Why mess with a great recipe? Put fruit on top of your Ryvita, not inside.	They beat even fatty Ritz Crackers into second place in the calorie race.	A staggering calorie level for one unflavoured cracker.	As a rule, steer clear of crackers with added flavour. It'll mess up your cheese, too.	These are buttery and puffy (the clue is in the name). So you get a big saturated fat hit.	Sweet stuff so the 2.2 g of sugar is no surprise. But 1 g of salt? Scary.

169

Dips

Eat This!

Doritos Nacho Cheese Dip
(⅓ jar, 100 g)

231 calories
20.2 g fat
(3.3 g saturated)
1 g salt

If you want a cheese dip Doritos get it right. You get your melted indulgence for 160 fewer calories than at Tesco

Discovery Guacamole
(⅓ bottle, 100 g)

79 calories
5.6 g fat
(3.5 g saturated)
1 g salt

A brilliant way to add avocado to your meal. Dip your nachos in it or add it to wraps. It's the best you'll find

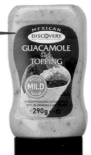

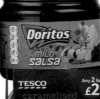

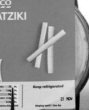

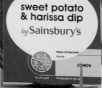

no artificial colours, flavours or preservatives added

Dairylea Dunkers
(1 pot, 47 g)

111 calories
3.9 g fat
(2.8 g saturated)
0.8 g salt

The pots are small for a reason. Stick to one and it's a decent snack. Two risks sat fat overload.

Tesco Tzatziki
(½ pot, 100 g)

145 calories
12 g fat
(4.5 g saturated)
0.5 g salt

Wherever you buy it from tzatziki is one of the best dips: yogurt and cucumber beat cream any day.

Doritos Mild Salsa
(⅔ jar, 100 g)

32.5 calories
trace fat
(trace saturated)
1.5 g salt

Doritos do it again with the lower calorie salsa dip than virtually any of their competitors.

Tesco Caramelised Onion Houmous
(½ pot, 100 g)

240 calories
19.4 g fat
(1.9 g saturated)
1.6 g salt

Houmous is always high in calories, but even with onions in it beats taramasalata.

Sainsbury's Sweet Potato & Harissa
(½ pot, 100 g)

93 calories
1.4 g fat
(0.2 g saturated)
0.64 g salt

Something unusual to keep party guests talking... without making them fat.

Not That!

Sainsbury's Guacamole
(½ pot, 100 g)

212 calories
20.2 g fat
(7.4 g saturated)
0.5 g salt

Most guacamole from supermarkets has a similar calorie count. Use sparingly or find a lighter version.

Dip with care if you find this cheesy one in front of you

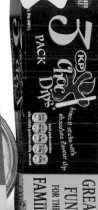

Tesco Nacho Cheese
(½ tub, 100 g)

390 calories
37.8 g fat
(3.5 g saturated)
0.8 g salt

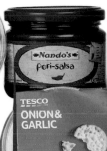

Sainsbury's Edamame & Wasabi
(½ pot, 100 g)

176 calories
13.8 g fat
(3.4 g saturated)
0.65 g salt

Another unusual dip. But one to avoid. It's not like anyone will be asking for it.

Tesco Taramasalata
(½ pot, 100 g)

515 calories
52.5 g fat
(3.5 g saturated)
1.2 g salt

Made with fish roe, just a few dips will tip the scales. Stick to other Greek specials houmous or tzatziki.

Nando's Peri Peri Salsa
(²⁄₅ jar, 100 g)

81 calories
0.5 g fat
(0.7 g saturated)
1.9 g salt

A calorie bonanza compared to similar salsas, no prizes for low salt levels either. Don't dip here.

Tesco Onion & Garlic
(½ pot, 100 g)

335 calories
33.3 g fat
(6.1 g saturated)
1 g salt

Sounds pretty healthy but there's so much cream in this, you'll get nearly a third of your day's sat fat.

KP Chocolate
(1 pot, 32 g)

170 calories
9.5 g fat
(3.4 g saturated)
0.1 g salt

No surprises here, having your dip made of chocolate isn't really a great idea. Even cheese is better.

171

Sauces & Dressings

Eat This!

Hellmann's Garlic Mayonnaise
(15 ml)
41 calories
4 g fat
(0.4 g saturated)
0.26 g salt

Flavoursome garlic means calories are cut dramatically. A brilliant way to get your mayo.

Daddies Tomato Ketchup
(100 g)
102 calories
trace fat
(trace saturate)
18.5 g sugar

Daddies wins in the battle of the sauces by cutting sugar content.

Oak Lane Caesar Dressing
(100 g)
220 calories
21.5 g fat
(2.1 g saturated)
4.4 g sugar

Caesar is a big-ticket sauce, but Oak Lane make it more acceptable.

Heinz Salad Cream with Lemon & Black Pepper
(100 g)
298 calories
23.3 g fat
(1.8 g saturated)
16.9 g sugar

Salad cream wins against mayonnaise.

Daddies Brown Sauce
(100 g)
108 calories
trace fat
(0 g saturated)
18.4 g sugar

Lower in sugar than bigger brand rival. Go for Daddies and you won't get bigger.

Newman's Own Ranch
(100 g)
278 calories
26.7 g fat
(2.1 g saturated)
3.9 g sugar

This ranch dressing is quite good… for a creamy dressing. Use with care.

Hellmann's Light Vinaigrette
(100 ml)
49 calories
0 g fat
(0 g saturated)
7.8 g sugar

Probably the best thing you can put on salad. Loads of flavour.

English Provider Co. Balsamic Italian Dressing
(100 g)
67 calories
2.7 fat
(0.5 g saturated)

Not even 'light' and still brilliant.

Branston Chilli & Jalapeno Relish
(100 g)
124 calories
0.7 g fat
(0 saturate)
24.4 g sugar

Not bad at all, although still high in sugar.

172

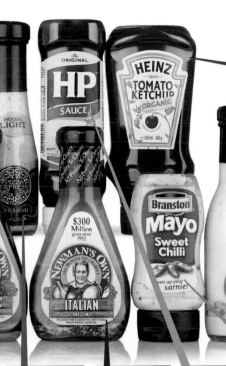

Hellmann's Real Mayonnaise
(15 ml)

100 calories
11 g fat
(0.9 g saturated)
0.2 g salt

Full-fat mayonnaise is never going to be a winner in the dressing stakes. Find an alternative.

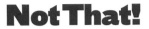

Not That!

Heinz Organic Tomato Ketchup
(100 g)

119 calories
trace fat
(trace saturated)
27 g sugar

Unfortunately organic doesn't mean low in calories or sugar

Tesco Caesar Dressing
(100 g)

270 calories
45.1 g fat
(3.2 g saturated)
4.6 sugar

You get 50 extra calories and more than twice the fat of the Oak Lane.

Tesco Onion Relish
(100 g)

145 calories
0.2 g fat
(trace saturate)
28.6 g sugar

Sweeter than it needs to be. You're better off with something a bit more spicy.

Newman's Own Balsamic
(100 g)

326 calories
33.3 g fat
(2 g saturated)
3 g sugar

In this match, England v America, We win... by 259 calories. Sorry, Paul Newman.

Pizza Express House Light
(100 ml)

297 calories
30.5 g fat
(4.6 g saturated)
3.3 g sugar

This is probably the worst 'light' product we've come across. It looks heavy to us.

Newman's Italian
(100 g)

649 calories
72.1 g fat
(6.6 g saturate)
0.2 g sugar

Italian dressing looks healthier than a creamy ranch. Beware. It's almost all oil.

HP Brown Sauce
(100 g)

122 calories
0.1 g fat
(trace saturate)
23.1 g sugar

Not a bad blob of sauce, but you can shave calories off with brands with a little less sugar.

Branston Sweet Chilli Mayo
(100 g)

477 calories
37.5 g fat
(2.8 g saturated)
1.75 g salt

Flavoured mayonnaise isn't always good. One to avoid.

173

Sausages

Eat This!

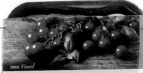

Tesco Finest Pork & Italian Cherry Tomato
(1 sausage)

120 calories
8.1g fat
(3.2g saturated)
0.7g salt

The luxury end of the sausage market doesn't have to mean piling on calories. Look for ones with added fruit or veg to keep fat levels under control.

Without the skin you get a smaller sausage, but also nearly 100 fewer calories PER sausage. Meet the saviour of the Full English

Wall's Skinless Pork
(1 sausage)

48 calories
6g fat
(3g saturated)
0.3g salt

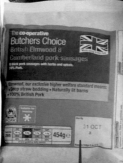

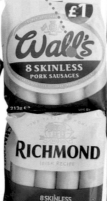

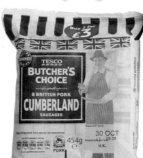

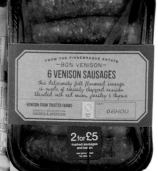

Tesco Butcher's Choice Cumberland
(1 sausage)

130 calories
8.5g fat
(3g saturated)
1.6g salt

A big saving of 40 calories and 2.5 g of saturated fat compared to a 'Finest' sausage.

Richmond Skinless
(1 sausage)

66 calories
5g fat
(2g saturated)
0.5g salt

Not to be outdone by their rivals Wall's, Richmond are in on the skinless act. They manage less fat, but 18 extra calories per banger.

Co-op Butchers Choice Cumberland
(1 sausage)

133 calories
9.5g fat
(3.4g saturated)
0.6g salt

In this case the Co-op butcher has made a reasonable choice, cutting calories and saturated fat compared to the high-end version.

Marks & Spencer Venison
(1 sausage)

95 calories
5.3g fat
(2.8g saturated)
0.75g salt

We crown venison king of sausages. These are 80% meat, so full of protein, but incredibly low in calories and fat. It doesn't get much better.

Tesco Finest Lincolnshire

(1 sausage)

185 calories
14.5 g fat
(5 g saturated)
0.75 g salt

Britain loses out to Italy in the Tesco Finest sausage stakes. Have three and get 75% of your saturated fat for the day. Not a great breakfast.

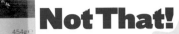

Not That!

Regularly opt for Wall's thickest sausage and you're asking for a thicker waistline

Wall's Thick Pork

(1 sausage)

136 calories
9 g fat
(4 g saturated)
1 g salt

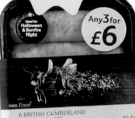

Any 3 for £6

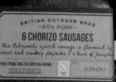

MIX & MATCH ANY 2 £5

new recipe

Marks & Spencer Chorizo

(1 sausage)

160 calories
12.9 g fat
(4.5 g saturated)
0.93 g salt

One of these is nearly twice as bad for your as the venison option. Steer clear of these Spanish waistline destroyers. Better eaten by the slice.

Co-op Truly Irresistilbe British Pork

(1 sausage)

163 calories
12.5 g fat
(4.1 g saturated)
0.6 g salt

With more meat, comes more fat and, curcially, more saturated fat. Tastier doesn't necessarily mean healthier.

Richmond Thick

(1 sausage)

125 calories
8 g fat
(4 g saturated)
1 g salt

Marginally healthier than the Wall's version, but this still has to fall on the unhealthy side of the sausage line when compared with the skinless variety.

Tesco Finest Cumberland Pork

(1 sausage)

170 calories
13 g fat
(5.5 g saturated)
150 mg sodium

You get around 10 g of protein per sausage. But the extra calories and sat fat mean your muscles aren't the only thing that will get filled out.

Soups

Eat This!

Tesco Finest Red Pepper Soup
(½ pot)

145 calories
6.3 g fat
(1.8 g saturated)
0.75 g salt

Opt for Tesco Finest Red Pepper for a hearty soup that's low in saturated fat.

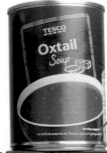

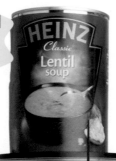

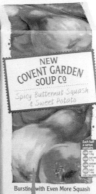

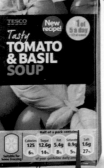

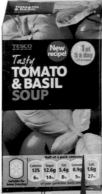

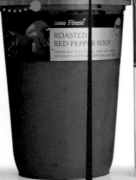

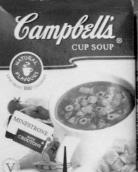

Tesco Tasty Tomato & Basil Soup
(½ carton)

125 calories
5.4 g fat
(0.9 saturated)
1.5 g salt

Tomato soups tend to be loaded with cream. This one cuts it out for less fat.

Heinz Classic Lentil Soup
(½ can)

93 calories
0.3 g fat
(0.1 g saturated)
1.25 g salt

This is quite simply one of the healthiest soups on the market, with virtually no fat in it at all.

Campbell's Minestrone Cup Soup
(1 sachet prepared)

86 calories
1.4 g fat
(0.6 g saturated)
1.13 g salt

Convenience and health in one box. Low in calories and fat. Stick the kettle on!

New Covent Garden Soup Co Squash & Sweet Potato
(½ carton)

120 calories
3.6 g fat
(2.1 g saturated)
1.35 g salt

A healthy, spicy winter soup to soothe the soul.

Not That!

Tesco Value Tomato Soup

(½ can)

95 calories
4 g fat
(0.2 g saturated)
0.4 g sodium

Not bad, but when compared to Tesco oxtail, the tomato comes off worse for calories and fat.

Tesco Finest Wild Mushroom Soup

(½ pot)

250 calories
17.1 g fat
(8.8 g saturated)
0.6 g sodium

This humble fungus broth hides nearly half of your saturated fat guideline daily amount.

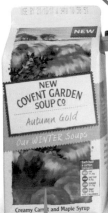

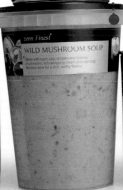

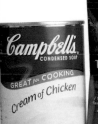

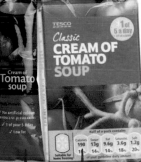

New Covent Garden Soup Co Autumn Gold

(½ carton)

177 calories
11.4 g fat
(6.9 g saturated)
2.25 g salt

This sneaks in double cream, butter and maple syrup for a high sat fat content.

Cambell's Condensed Soup Cream of Chicken

(½ can prepared)

149 calories
10 g fat
(1.2 g saturated)
1.68 g salt

Even when you thin it down, this still packs a calorie punch.

Heinz Squeeze & Stir Cream of Tomato Soup

(1 cup prepared)

144 calories
7.2 g fat
(0.6 g saturated)
1.5 g salt

Not a disastrous cup of soup, but there are better products on the market.

Tesco Classic Cream Of Tomato Soup

(½ carton)

190 calories
9.6 g fat
(3.6 saturated)
1.5 g sodium

It's not just the cream driving up calories here—it's also a glut of added sugar.

177

Yogurt

Eat This!

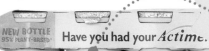

Have you had your *Actimel*

The probiotic yogurt market has exploded in recent years. Make sure your waistline doesn't too with these.

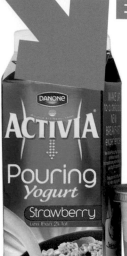

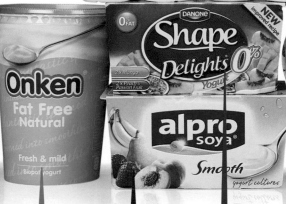

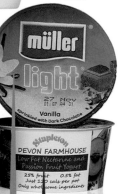

NEW BOTTLE
95% PLANT-BASED

Acitiva Pouring Yogurt (100 g)	**Onken Fat Free Natural** (100 g)	**Alpro Soya** (1 pot, 125 g)	**Shape Delights** (peach) (1 pot, 120 g)	**Müller Light Vanilla & Chocolate** (100 g)	**Stapleton Nectarine & Passionfruit** (100 g)
56 calories 1.6 g fat (1 g saturated) 7.2 g sugar	48 calories 0.1 g fat (0.1 g saturated) 6.3 g sugar	95 calories 2.4 g fat (0.4 g saturated) 13 g sugar	80 calories 0.1 g fat (0.1 g saturated) 9.3 g sugar	55 calories 0.5 g fat (0.3 g saturated) 7.1 g sugar	80 calories 0.5 g fat (0.3 g saturated) 16.3 g sugar
A convenient way to drink yoghurt that keeps sugar content low.	When buying any brand of natural yogurt fat free is the way to go.	A little soya goes a long way in this pot that keeps fat low, without shouting about it.	Impressively low in fat, sugar levels aren't too bad either. A top pot.	A chocolate dessert that's as healthy as they come	Luxury yogurt that doesn't break the calorie or fat bank. Genius.

Not That!

Muller Vitality
(1 pot, 100 g)
72 calories
1.4 g fat
(0.9 g saturated)
11.2 g sugar

These have more than twice the calories of Actimel and more fat, despite claiming to be low in the stuff.

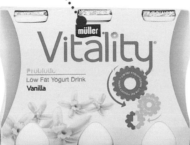

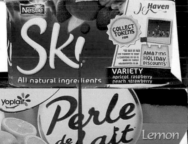

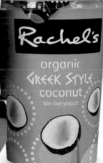

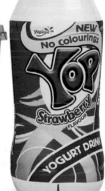

Collective Dairy Passionfruit
(100 g)
140 calories
5 g fat
(3.1 g saturated)
18.1 g sugar

Sugary fruit syrup combine with fat-laden yogurt. A losing team.

Müller Amore Walnut & Honey
(100 g)
160 calories
8.7 g fat
(5 g saturated)
16.4 g sugar

All dials turned to indulgent. This more pudding than yogurt.

Ski Variety
(1 pot, 120 g)
113 calories
3.1 g fat
(2 g saturated)
15.1 g sugar

There's a fair amount of sugar and fat here, especially for a non-luxury brand. A basic best avoided.

Yoplait Perle De Lait Lemon
(1 pot, 125 g)
179 calories
10.8 g fat
(7.2 g saturated)
14.3 g sugar

Lemons have a reputation for being 'light'. Not in the case of this.

Rachel's Organic Greek Style Yogurt
(100 g)
156 calories
11.1 g fat
(7 g saturated)
10.1 g sugar

The lesson? Go low-fat and skip flavours in Greek.

Yop Drinking Yogurt
(100 g)
77 calories
1.3 g fat
(0.3 g saturated)
12.7 g sugar

Yop corner the fat end of the yogurt drink market, but only just.

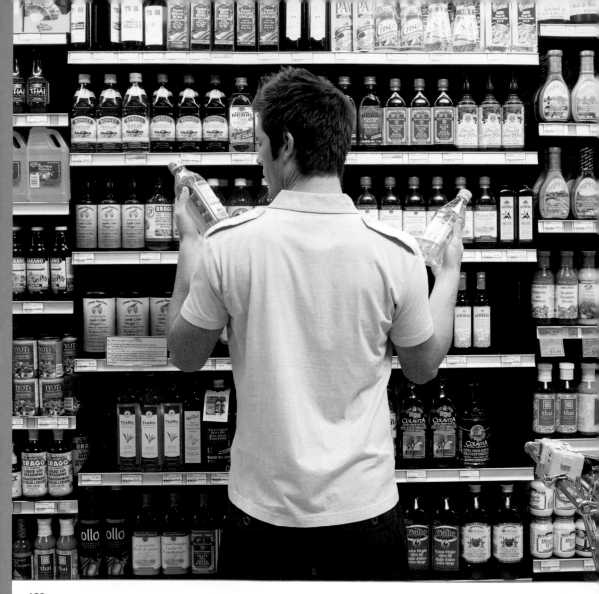

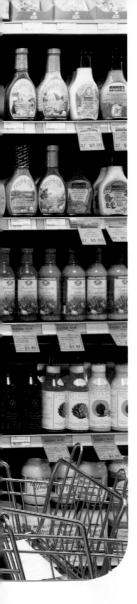

Main Courses

Whether you're taking care of yourself or a family of six, this handy section will show you how to pick the least calorific dinners from the shelf

Look out for our star picks on each page. The comparison may astound you. Who knew two similar products could be so different?

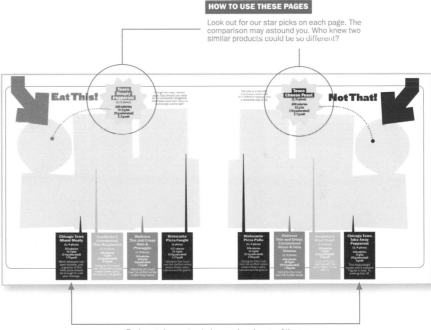

Eat This!

Tesco Simply Pepperoni
(1/3 pizza)
400 calories
19.5g fat
(9g saturated)
2.3g salt

Although this salty cheese laden food should only really be an occasional indulgent, this cheesy pizza from Tesco is surprisingly calorie-light.

The clue is in the title. This cheese-covered and more different choices can have a whopping 22g of fat.

Tesco Cheese Feast
(1/2 pizza)
650 calories
32g fat
(18g saturated)
2.7g salt

Not That!

Chicago Town Miami Meaty
(1/4 pizza)
315 calories
15.7g fat
(7.4g saturated)
1.7g salt

While deep-pan can spell disaster, just a quarter of this hefty pizza should be enough to curb your cravings.

Goodfella's Stonebaked Thin Margherita
(1/2 pizza)
356 calories
17g fat
(6.9g saturated)
1.5g salt

Opting for thin and crisp over the stuffed variety means fewer calories and fat grams.

Waitrose Thin and Crispy Ham & Pineapple
(1/2 pizza)
363 calories
16.9g fat
(6g saturated)
1.7g salt

Ristorante Pizza Funghi
(1 pizza)
427 calories
18.4g fat
(8.8g saturated)
2.27g salt

Opting for thin crust over the stuffed variety means fewer carbs, calories and fat grams.

Ristorante Pizza Pollo
(1/2 pizza)
576 calories
16.7g fat
(5.5g saturated)
2.98g salt

Opting for thin crust over the stuffed means fewer carbs, calories and fat grams.

Waitrose Thin and Crispy Caramelised Onion & Feta Cheese
(1/2 pizza)
614 calories
30.6g fat
(13.5g saturated)
1.3g salt

Opting for thin crust over the stuffed variety means...

Goodfella's Stuffed Feast
(1/4 pizza)
615 calories
30g fat
(14.5g saturated)
1.6g salt

Chicago Town Take Away Pepperoni
(1/4 pizza)
654 calories
35g fat
(16g saturated)
3g salt

This heavyweight comes with a massive 70g fat in total. Try kicking that off.

Each page is constructed as a mirror image of the one opposite. Compare similar products on each side by reading the same coloured boxes on both pages.

Red Meat

Eat This!

Sainsbury's Taste the Difference Lamb Moussaka
(½ pack)

480 calories
12 g fat
(6.5 g saturated)

The tomatoes and aubergine in this more fat-friendly moussaka will fill you up without the added calories of the Tesco equivalent

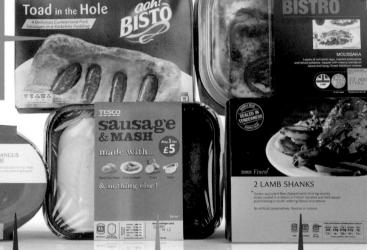

Bisto Toad in the Hole
(½ pack, 150 g)

347 calories
11.3 g fat
(2.1 g saturated)
1.1 g salt

Essentially just sausages in batter, this may not be your healthiest dinner but its low sat-fat content means it's not the worst dish on offer.

Tesco Finest Aberdeen Angus Cottage Pie
(1 pack, 430 g)

440 calories
18.6 g fat
(7 g saturated)
3.1 g salt

Made with British beef, and a splash of red wine, this cottage pie will fill you up without filling you out.

Tesco Sausage and Mash
(1 pack, 450 g)

480 calories
21 g fat
(7 g saturated)
2.4 g salt

Bangers and mash may get a bad rep, but this option (complete with onion gravy) is relatively low in calories and sat fats.

Tesco Finest Lamb Shank
(1 shank, 425 g)

334 calories
18 g fat
(8 g saturated)
1 g salt

The flavour here comes from the seven varieties of herb found in these shanks—and you're looking at a decent dose of protein, too.

This hefty meal comes with over three times the fat content of Sainsbury's lighter option. Scoff the lot and you're looking at almost 1,200 calories

Not That!

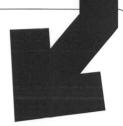

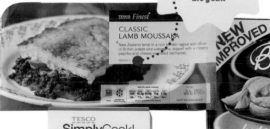

Tesco Finest Lamb Moussaka
(1/2 pack)
580 calories
43 g fat
(15 g saturated)
2.5 g salt

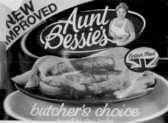

Aunt Bessie's Toad in the Hole
(1 pack 190 g)
437 calories
20.9 g fat
(4.2 g saturated)
1.8 g salt

It may be butcher's choice, but it's not ours. By swapping Bessie's for a serving of Bisto you can save yourself nearly 100 calories.

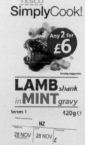

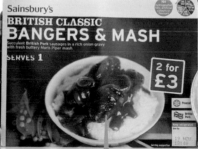

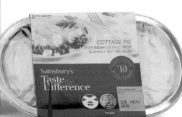

Tesco Lamb Shank with Mint Gravy
(1 shank, 420 g)
515 calories
26 g fat
(12 g saturated)
2.3 g salt

A sprig of mint can be a healthy addition to lamb dishes—the problem here is the caramelised sugar syrup used to make this gravy.

Sainsbury's Bangers and Mash
(1 meal, 450 g)
662 calories
34.9 g fat
(19.8 g saturated)
2.2 g salt

With the high fat content in this porky offering from Sainsbury's, you're better off donning an apron and digging out the potato peeler.

Sainsbury's Taste The Difference Cottage Pie
(1 package, 400 g)
581 calories
27.7 g fat
(16.2 g saturated)
2.5 g salt

Although 30 grams lighter this pie packs 141 extra calories compared to Tesco's leaner option.

Chicken

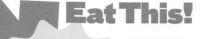

Eat This!

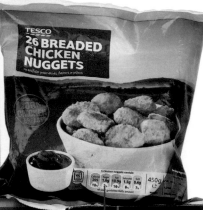

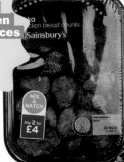

Sainsbury's Cooked Chicken Tikka Breast pieces

(100 g)

129 calories
1.8 g fat
(0.4 g saturated)
0.78 g salt

Stick to chicken breast for a leaner cut however it's prepared.

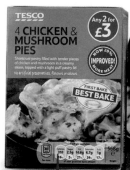

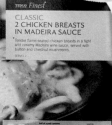

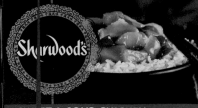

Tesco Chicken & Mushroom Pies

(1 pie, 142 g)

310 calories
15 g fat
(7 g saturated)
1 g salt

Chicken goes well with mushroom and as they're one of the only vegetables to contain vitamin D, this is a fine compliment to your pie.

Tesco Finest Chicken with Mushrooms & Madeira Sauce

(1 serving)

220 calories
8 g fat
(3 g saturated)
1.7 g salt

Even covered in a creamy sauce the fat content is low. A good cheesy pasta hit.

Tesco Breaded Chicken Nuggets

(5 nuggets)

205 calories
10.9 g fat
(2 g saturated)
0.4 g salt

The value here is for just 5 nuggets, so make sure to regulate how many fall on to your, or your child's, plate.

Sharwood's Sweet and Sour Chicken

(1 serving)

480 calories
4.5 g fat
(1 g saturated)
1.8 g salt

Keep things sweet and cut the fat in half by opting for this dish over most supermarket own brands.

Not That!

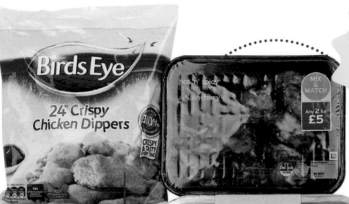

(½ pack)
(100 g)
241 calories
15.7 g fat
(3.5 g saturated)
1.14 g salt

Chicken wings aren't the super food that breast is. They're fatty and calorific, plus you don't even get much meat on each one.

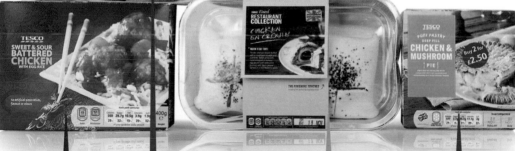

Tesco Sweet & Sour Chicken

(1 serving)

560 calories
11 g fat
(4 g saturated)
1.9 g salt

You'll be left feeling sour if you ingest the 5 extra grams of fat in this compared to the lighter option of the same Chinese classic.

Birds Eye Crispy Chicken Dippers

(5 dippers)

215 calories
12 g fat
(2 g saturated)
0.9 g salt

Dippers are a shade worse than nuggets. There's not much in it but one had to lose the nutritional stand off.

Tesco Restaurant Collection Chicken En Croute

(1 serving)

645 calories
36 g fat
(16 g saturated)
2.3 g salt

Restaurant levels of calories in this meal. And that's before you even consider serving it with a side dish.

Tesco Deep Filled Chicken & Mushroom Pie

(1 pie, 234 g)

577 calories
36 g fat
(18 g saturated)
2 g salt

Deep filled apparently means stuffing in more calories and rich fatty sauce. Dig a little deeper for your pie choice.

185

Curry

Eat This!

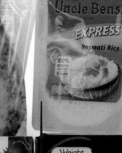

Tesco Garlic & Coriander Naan
(1 naan, 160 g)
425 calories
8 g fat
(1.4 g saturated)
1.3 g salt

A big calorie hit, but garlic and herbs cut the fat count. Added flavour and less fat? A double win.

Sainsbury's Chicken Jalfrezi
(½ pack, 200 g)
214 calories
10.7 g fat
(0.8 g saturated)
0.98 g salt

Even if you munch the whole thing that's still only 428 calories to burn off.

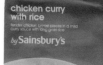

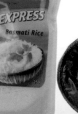

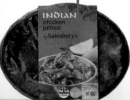

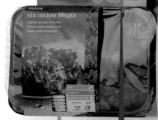

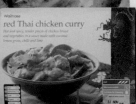

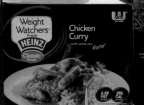

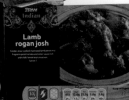

Waitrose Onion Bhajis
(1 bhaji)
103 calories
7 g fat
(0.6 g saturated)
0.4 g salt

At 100 calories each, these are indulgent but beat the samosa as your Indian starter.

Sainsbury's Chicken Curry with Rice
(1 pack, 400 g)
456 calories
8.7 g fat
(4.4 g saturated)
2.1 g salt

A little bit salty, but a lot less calories than its beef counterpart.

Waitrose Red Thai Curry
(1 pack, 350 g)
358 calories
20.6 g fat
(10.8 g saturated)
2.6 g salt

A low calorie count, but eyes open for the half your GDA of saturated fat.

Uncle Ben's Express Basmati Rice
(1 serving, 125 g)
191 calories
2 g fat
(0.3 g saturated)
0.22 g salt

White is right when it comes to this rice stand off. But brown is better.

Weight Watchers Chicken Curry
(1 pack, 320 g)
301 calories
4.5 g fat
(1.1 g saturated)
1.6 g salt

Only 300 calories puts this curry in a league of it's own.

Tesco Rogan Josh
(1 pack, 350 g)
415 calories
21.7 g fat
(5.8 g saturated)
2.4 g salt

Spicier on the palate but easier on your waistline compared to the Korma.

186

Not That!

Sainsbury's Chicken Tikka Masala
(½ pack, 200 g)

326 calories
20.1 g fat
(7.9 g saturated)
1.2 g salt

Stick to the half pack guidelines or you're in for a 40 gram fat attack.

Without any flavouring this naan relies on extra butter to tickle your tastebuds. Go for garlic instead.

Tesco Plain Naan
1 naan, 160 g

425 calories
11.7 g fat
(2.9 g saturated)
1.3 g salt

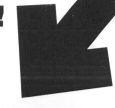

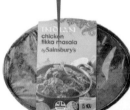

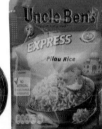

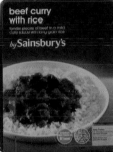

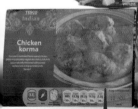

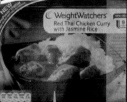

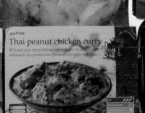

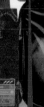

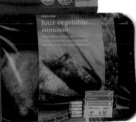

Tesco Chicken Korma
(1 pack, 350 g)

610 calories
38.2 g fat
(14 g saturated)
2.3 g salt

It may be famously mild in spice, but not so in the dieting department

Weight Watchers Red Thai Curry
(1 pack, 400 g)

342 calories
3.2 g fat
(1.6 g saturated)
2.09 g salt

If you're going for Weight Watchers curry, opt for the simple chicken.

Uncle Ben's Express Pilau Rice
(1 serving, 125 g)

214 calories
4.4 g fat
(0.6 g saturated)
0.56 g salt

Steamed with sunflower oil, just not enough to be of any benefit to you.

Waitrose Thai Peanut Curry
(1 pack, 350g)

462 calories
25.5 g fat
(7 g saturated)
0.94 g salt

A few peanuts add up on the calorie calculator in this dish.

Sainsbury's Beef Curry with Rice
(1 pack, 400g)

508 calories
10.4 g fat
(4.4 g saturated)
2.1 g salt

This beefs up the calorie intake for curry lovers.

Waitrose Vegetable Samosa
(1 samosa)

123 calories
7.5 g fat
(0.66 g saturated)
0.56 g salt

Not all vegetable concoctions are good for you. Don't over indulge here.

Fish

Eat This!

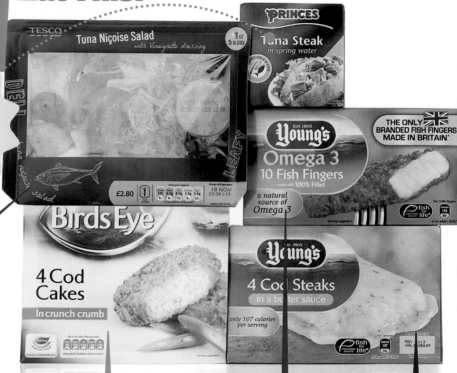

Princes Tuna Steak in Spring Water
(100 g)
105 calories
0.5 g fat
(trace saturated)
0.75 g salt

No oils means a virtually fat free tuna for you.

PRINCES
Tuna Steak
in spring water

TESCO
Tuna Niçoise Salad
with Vinaigrette dressing

£2.80

Young's
Est. 1805
Omega 3
10 Fish Fingers
made with 100% Fillet
a natural source of Omega 3

THE ONLY BRANDED FISH FINGERS MADE IN BRITAIN*

Birds Eye
4 Cod Cakes
In crunch crumb

Young's
Est. 1805
4 Cod Steaks
in a butter sauce
only 107 calories per serving

Tesco Tuna Nicoise Salad
(meal, 210g)
175 calories
8.7 g fat
(1.1 g saturated)
1.1 g salt

Complete with whole cherry tomatoes and new potatoes, this is a great mix of nutrition for a salad.

Birds Eye Cod Fish Cakes
(2 cakes)
185 calories
8 g fat
(1 g saturated)
1 g salt

These are a little smaller than the Young's version but you can double up and still save yourself a few calories and a couple of grams of fat.

Young's Omega 3 Fish Fingers
(3 fingers, 84g)
160 calories
8.5 g fat
(0.9 g saturated)
0.5 g salt

There is so much goodness in the right fish, even in finger form. Do yourself a favour and ditch the chips for a fish finger sandwich.

Young's Cod Steaks in Butter Sauce
(per serving)
107 calories
3 g fat
(2 g saturated)
1 g salt

Butter sauce? Doesn't sound like a good idea, but these unbattered fish steaks are a welcome addition to the table.

Not That!

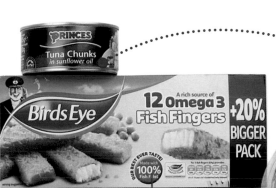

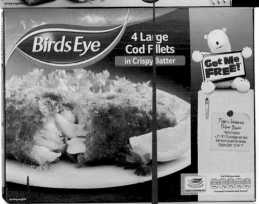

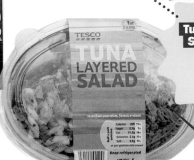

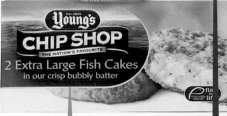

Pinces Tuna Chunks in Sunflower Oil
(100 g)

197 calories
10.8 g fat
(2 g saturated)
0.8 g salt

There are good things about sunflower oil. But cutting calories isn't one.

Bird's Eye Large Cod Fillets in Batter
(per serving)

315 calories
19 g fat
(2.4 g saturated)
1.4 g salt

A breadcrumb coating will workout slightly healthier than this batter. But you're better off going with none at all.

Bird's Eye Omega 3 Fish Fingers
(100 g)

220 calories
9.3 g fat
(1.1 g saturated)
0.9 g salt

Gram for gram Bird's Eye still have 10% more calories than the Young's version. So you can pass on that invitation to the Captain's table.

Young's Chip Shop Fish Cakes
(1 cake)

216 calories
10.6 g fat
(2.3 g saturated)
1 g salt

Only 32 percent fish and 8 percent diced potato, leaves 60 percent to be made up by the other 25 ingredients.

Tesco Tuna Layered Salad Bowl
(½ pack, 190 g)

220 calories
11 g fat
(2 g saturated)
0.8 g salt

A bit of veg but that pasta piles on the carbohydrates sending this into the salad danger zone.

Pasta

Eat This!

Trattoria Verdi Potato Gnocchi
(125 g)

190 calories
0.6 g fat
(0 g saturated)
1.3 g salt

You'd think potato in pasta would be a no-no, but stick to one portion and it's a winner.

Sainsbury's Basics Spaghetti Bolognese
(1 pack, 300 g)

301 calories
5.9 g fat
(2.6 g saturated)
1.17 g salt

A brilliant basic meal, ready in a few minutes in the microwave and doesn't go overboard on any of the bad stuff.

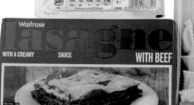

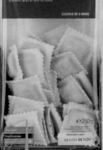

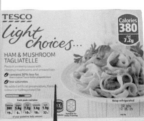

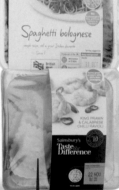

Waitrose Lasagne With Beef
(½ pack, 350 g)

367 calories
16.8 g fat
(8.6 g saturated)
1.86 g salt

Share with a friend and the smaller portion size means this beats the 'healthy' version (opposite) on calories and salt.

Waitrose Cheese, Tomato and Basil Ravioli
(½ pack, 125 g)

271 calories
9 g fat
(5.5 g saturated)
0.59 g salt

Admirably low in calories and fat, especially considering the cheese content. A healthy way to get your cheesy pasta hit.

Tesco Light Choices Ham And Mushroom Tagliatelle
(1 pack, 400 g)

380 calories
7 g fat
(4 g saturated)
1.9 g salt

A creamy pasta treat, that keeps the calories under control as well as giving you a big portion size. Brilliant.

Sainsbury's Taste The Difference King Prawn & Chilli Ravioli
(½ pack, 125 g)

299 calories
9.8 g fat
(3.8 g saturated)
1.54 g salt

A rich treat that won't fill you out (if you stick to the suggested half a pack) so make sure you share

Not That!

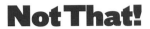

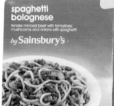

Sainsbury's Spaghetti Bolognese
(frozen)
(1 pack, 400 g)
382 calories, 4.3 g fat
(2 g saturated)
1.28 g salt

Not bad, but for some reason you get 100 g more Bolognese from Sainsbury's when you buy it frozen. Go for the fresh option for portion control.

Tesco Tagliatelle
(75 g)
270 calories
1.1 g fat
(0.2 g saturated)
0 g salt

Traditional pasta has a deserved reputation for adding calories to your meal.

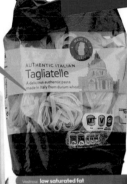

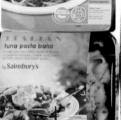

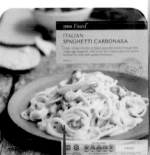

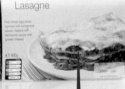

Sainsbry's Italian Tuna Pasta Bake
(1 pack, 400 g)
601 calories
24.3 g fat
(14.5 g saturated)
1.67 g salt

You do get 31.7 g of protein from the tuna, but the fat levels mean there are much healthier ways to build muscle.

Tesco Finest Spaghetti Carbonara
(1 pack, 400 g)
890 calories
53 g fat
(27 g saturated)
2 g salt

It may have the finest taste but your body won't thank you in the long run. Taking on 133% of your GDA of sat fat in one dish is pushing it.

Waitrose Prosciutto & Cheese Cappelletti
(½ pack, 125 g)
364 calories
9.3 g fat
(3 g saturated)
0.88 g salt

Over 90 extra calories per portion compared to ravioli (opposite). Eat the whole pack and it's like having the ravioli with a bag of Maltesers.

Waitrose Low Saturated Fat Lasagne
(1 packet, 400g)
388 calories
10.4 g fat
(4.4 g saturated)
1.95 g salt

This is admirably low in saturates, but the calorie and salt counts are higher than the regular version (opposite).

191

Pizza

Eat This!

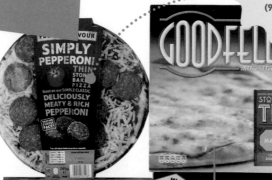

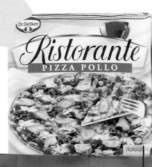

Tesco Simply Pepperoni
(½ pizza)
400 calories
19.5 g fat
(9 g saturated)
2.3 g salt

By opting for a thinner base you can have a meaty pizza from Tesco and it'll still be surprisingly calorie-light.

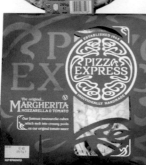

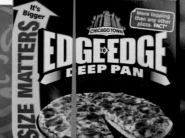

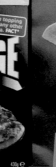

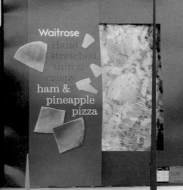

Pizza Express Margherita (½ pizza)	**Chicago Town Miami Meaty** (¾ pizza)	**Goodfella's Stonebaked Thin Margherita** (¼ pizza)	**Waitrose Thin and Crispy Ham & Pineapple** (⅓ pizza)	**Ristorante Pizza Pollo** (½ pizza)
260 calories 7.1 g fat (4.2 g saturated) 1.2 g salt	311 calories 15.7 g fat (7.4 g saturated) 1.75 g salt	256 calories 11 g fat (5.2 g saturated) 0.9 g salt	343 calories 10.9 g fat (4 g saturated) 1.5 g salt	378 calories 16.3 g fat (5.5 g saturated) 2.05 g salt
This please-all pizza is low calories, so you could work the whole thing off in one gym session.	While deep-pan can spell disaster, this is considerably lower in calories than the 'Takeaway' version.	Opting for thin crust over the deep variety means fewer carbs, calories and fat.	Surprisingly way better than the veggie version.	A colourful creation and frozen veg can retains its nutritional values. On a pizza or otherwise.

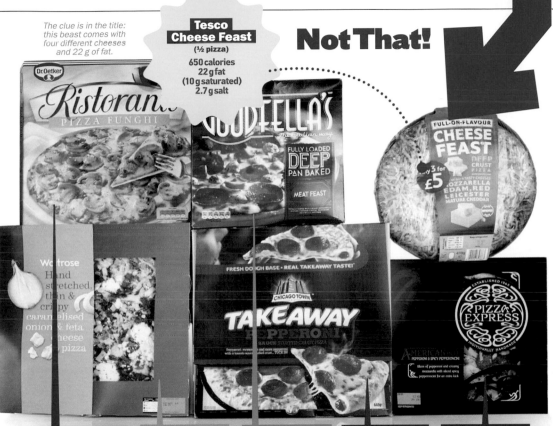

The clue is in the title: this beast comes with four different cheeses and 22 g of fat.

Tesco Cheese Feast
(½ pizza)
650 calories
22 g fat
(10 g saturated)
2.7 g salt

Not That!

FULL-ON-FLAVOUR
CHEESE FEAST
DEEP CRUST PIZZA
MOZZARELLA, EDAM, RED LEICESTER, MATURE CHEDDAR
Any 3 for £5

Ristorante Pizza Funghi
(½ pizza)

427 calories
22.4 g fat
(5.8 g saturated)
2.27 g salt

This pizza has caramelised sugar in it, maybe they are trying to keep customers sweet.

Waitrose Thin and Crispy Caramelised Onion & Feta Cheese
(1/3 pizza)

446 calories
20.8 g fat
(10.9 g saturated)
1.36 g salt

Even thin and crispy can offend.

Goodella's Meat Feast
(¼ pizza)

312 calories
13 g fat
(5.6 g saturated)
1.3 g salt

A rule of thumb: Anything with the word "feast" in the title is usually calorific.

Chicago Town Take Away Pepperoni
(¼ pizza)

446 calories
19 g fat
(10 g saturated)
3 g salt

This heavyweight comes with a massive 76g fat in total. Try working that off.

Pizza Express American Hot
(½ pizza)

305 calories
11.3 g fat
(5.2 g saturated)
1.85 g salt

Unsurprisingly, the addition of fatty meat to this pizza does it no favours in the calorie department.

193

Potatoes

Eat This!

When you've no time to home-mash, then homestyle is the next best option

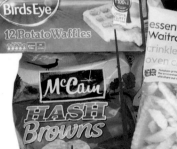

Not That!

Sainsbury's Taste The Difference Maris Piper Mash

(100 g)

135 calories,
8.3 g fat
(5.4 g saturated)
0.48 g salt

McCain Crispy French Fries

(100 g)

270 calories
10.9 g fat
(1.4 g saturated)
1 g salt

With well over 200 calories a serving, these fries are best avoided.

The more buttery your mash, the more it will expand your waistline.

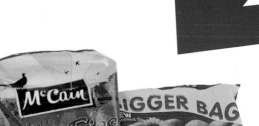

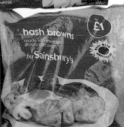

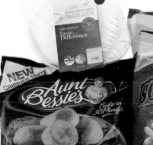

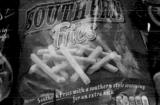

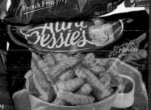

Aunt Bessie's Crispy Roast Potatoes

(100 g)

167 calories
5.8 g fat
(2.7 g saturated)
0.5 g salt

These Sunday roast staples come lightly battered—it's better to make your own.

McCain Southern Fries

(100 g)

228 calories
8.5 g fat
(1 g saturated)
0.6 g salt

These fries are thin, but with 8.5 grams of fat per 100 they're unlikely to have the same effect on you.

Aunt Bessie's Crinkle Cut Chips

(100 g)

212 calories
9.2 g fat
(4.5 g saturated)
0.2 g salt

A serving of these comes with 76 more calories than the Waitrose equivalent.

McCain Smiles

(100 g)

215 calories
8.8 g fat
(1 g saturated)
0.2 g salt

We're not sure what McCain are smiling about. These cheerful chips lose out to the good old-fashioned waffle .

Sainsbury's Hash Browns

(100 g)

205 calories
10 g fat
(1.1 g saturated)
0.75 g salt

A little more oil bumps up the fat content and the calories along with it.

Vegetarian

Eat This!

Linda McCartney Vegetarian Cannelloni

(1 pack, 375 g)

386 calories
12.8 g fat
(6.4 g saturated)
2 g salt

With a modest calorie content and half the fat of the Tesco's version, all you need is McCartney.

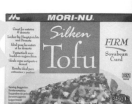

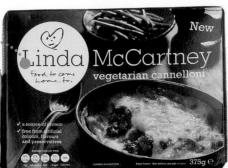

New

Linda McCartney
vegetarian cannelloni

Food to come home to.

✓ a source of protein
✓ free from artificial colours, flavours and preservatives

375g ℮

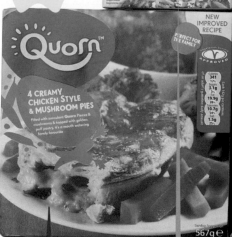

Quorn™

4 CREAMY CHICKEN STYLE & MUSHROOM PIES

Filled with succulent Quorn Pieces & mushrooms & topped with golden puff pastry. It's a mouth watering family favourite.

NEW IMPROVED RECIPE

567g ℮

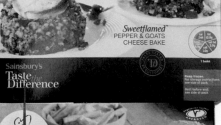

Sweetflamed™
PEPPER & GOATS CHEESE BAKE

Sainsbury's
Taste the Difference

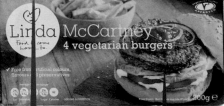

Linda McCartney
4 vegetarian burgers

Food to come home to.

✓ Free from artificial colours, flavours and preservatives

500g ℮

Quorn Creamy Chicken Style & Mushroom Pies

(1 pie, 142 g)

341 calories
20 g fat
(11 g saturated)
1.5 g salt

Portion control in action. A slightly smaller pie means you'll save 100 calories over McCartney's version.

Mori-Nu Silken Tofu

(100 g)

62 calories
3 g fat

Light on calories while still full of protein, this silken tofu can be blended into soups and smoothies or even 'scrambled' with a handful of veg as an egg alternative.

Sainsbury's Taste The Difference Sweetflamed Pepper & Goat's Cheese Bake

(½ pack, 140 g)

244 calories
10.8 g fat
(3.9 g saturated)
1 g salt

A way for cheese-addicts to get their fix, without going too heavy on the sat fats.

Linda McCartney Vegetarian Burgers

(1 burger, 50 g)

64 calories
1.5 g fat
(0.5 g saturated)
0.4 g salt

Great for veggies after protein, or even for meat-eaters trying to shift fat. The low levels of sat fat make these burgers a winner.

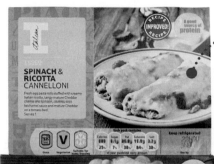

SPINACH & RICOTTA CANNELLONI

Fresh egg pasta rolls stuffed with creamy Italian ricotta, tangy mature Cheddar cheese and spinach, covered with a béchamel sauce and mature Cheddar on a tomato bed. Serves 1

Not That!

Tesco Spinach & Ricotta Cannelloni
(1 pack, 400 g)

508 calories
27 g fat
(17 g saturated)
2.3 g salt

With almost 30g of fat, the healthy spinach here is overruled by the cream and cheese used to pad out this pasta dish.

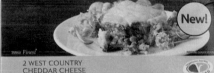

New!

2 WEST COUNTRY CHEDDAR CHEESE & FOUR NUT ROASTS
280g

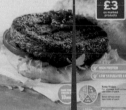

love **soya**

2 meatfree quarter pounders
with a chargrilled finish

by **Sainsbury's**

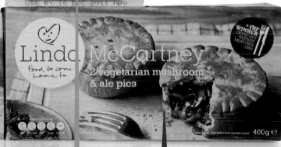

Any 2 for £3

Linda McCartney
Food to come home to.
2 vegetarian mushroom & ale pies
400g ℮

Sainsbury's Meatfree Quarter Pounders
(1 burger, 113.5 g)

178 calories
7.4 g fat
(1.2 g saturated)
1.44 g salt

Twice the size of the McCartney burgers but with almost five times the fat content per burger. Best stick to the lighter variety.

Tesco Finest West Country Cheddar & Four Nut Roasts
(1 roast, 135 g)

420 calories
27 g fat
(10 g saturated)
1.2 g salt

Nut roasts can be a good source of meat-free protein, but hold back on the cheddar if you're counting calories.

Cauldron Tofu
(100 g)

85 calories
4.2 g fat

While still a low-fat, natural option, Cauldron's tofu is higher in calories than Mori-Nu's and comes in a slightly bigger pack, so you'll be likely to eat more.

Linda McCartney Mushroom & Ale Pies
(1 pie, 200 g)

439 calories
23.5 g fat
(10.2 g saturated)
1.3 g salt

Hefty pies with a hefty caloric count. Delicious, perhaps, but they won't help you win in the battle of the bulge.

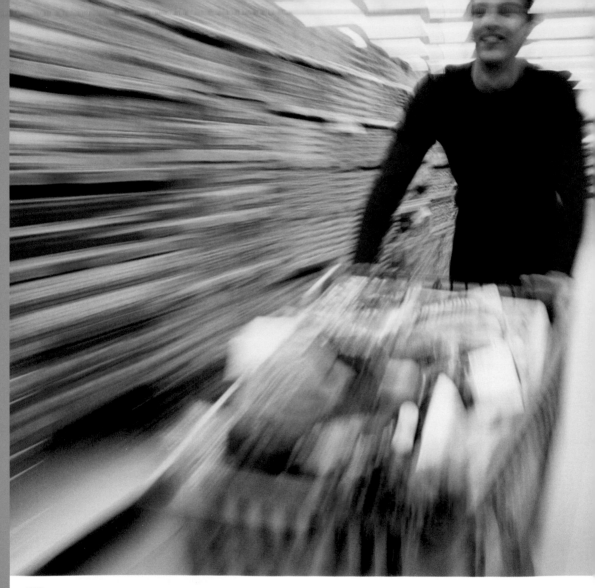

Treats

You don't have to leave sweet stuff out of your trolley. Follow our advice and you will be surprised at how much you can indulge

HOW TO USE THESE PAGES

Look out for our star picks on each page. The comparison may astound you. Who knew two similar products could be so different?

Eat This!

Tesco Simply Pepperoni
(1/4 pizza)
400 calories
19.3g fat
(9 g saturated)
2.3g salt

Not That!

Tesco Cheese Feast
(1/2 pizza)
600 calories
22g fat
(10 g saturated)
2.7g salt

Chicago Town Miami Meaty (1/4 pizza)	GoodFella's Stonebaked Thin Margherita (1/4 pizza)	Waitrose Thin and Crispy Ham & Pineapple (1/3 pizza)	Ristorante Pizza Funghi (1 pizza)	Ristorante Pizza Pollo (1 pizza)	Waitrose Thin and Crispy Onion & Feta Cheese (1/3 pizza)	Goodfella's Meat Feast (1/4 pizza)	Chicago Town Take Away Pepperoni (1/4 pizza)

Each page is constructed as a mirror image of the one opposite. Compare similar products on each side by reading the same coloured boxes on both pages.

Biscuits

Eat This!

Maryland Choc Chip

(1 biscuit)

51 calories
2.4 g fat
(1.2 g saturated)
3.9 g sugar

A better option due to it's size, stick to one and it can be a better biscuit than most.

Fox's Creams Rich Tea

53 calories
2.5 g fat
(1.4 g saturated)
3.3 g sugar

If you're after a cream-filled treat, take this biscuit.

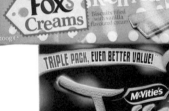

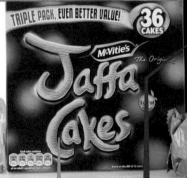

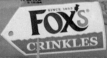

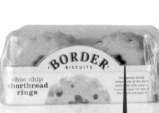

Border Chocolate Chip Shortbread

(1 biscuit)

75 calories
4.1 g fat
(2.5 g saturated)
3.3 g sugar

Choc chip undercut their fruit alternative.

McVities Jaffa Cakes

(1 cake)

46 calories
1 g fat
(0.5 g saturated)
6.4 g sugar

A higher sugar content due to it's natural fructose. It's still a lighter option, though.

McVitie's Rich Tea

(1 biscuit)

38 calories
1.3 g fat
(0.1 g saturated)
1.7 g sugar

In moderation the Rich Tea is the best biscuit to dunk in your cuppa.

Fox's Crinkles

(1 biscuit)

48 calories
1.4 g fat
(0.7 g saturated)
4.3 g sugar

Half the fat and sat fat of the crunch creams opposite. A much better option.

McVities Chocolate Digestive

(1 biscuit)

84 calories
4 g fat
(2.1 g saturated)
5.1 g sugar

Not the worst chocolate biscuit but needs to be an occasional treat.

McVitie's Digestives

(1 biscuit)

70 calories
3 g fat
(trace saturate)
3 g sugar

The classic falls on the wrong side due to it's larger size and 70 calories per munch waistline cost.

Not That!

Fox's Golden Crunch Creams

(1 biscuit)

79 calories
3.9 g fat
(2.3 g saturated)
6 g sugar

Fox's also do a cream-filled biscuit that's best avoided if you're watching the calories.

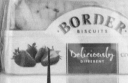

McVities Chocolate Hobnobs

(1 biscuit)

95 calories
5 g fat
(2 g saturated)
6 g sugar

How to make a hobnob worse for you? Add chocolate.

Fox's Ginger Crunch Cream

(1 biscuit)

78 calories
3.8 g fat
(2.2 g saturated)
6.3 g sugar

Double the layers, double the calories.

McVitie's Hobnobs

(1 biscuit)

73 calories
3 g fat
(trace saturate)
4 g sugar

With or without a chocolate top this falls on to the wrong side of the nutritional tracks.

Maryland Big & Chunky

(1 biscuit)

131 calories
7 g fat
(4 g saturated)
8 g sugar

Five provide your full GDA of sat fat and the calorie equivalent of most ready meals.

Border Strawberry & Current Shortbread

(1 biscuit)

85 calories
5 g fat
(3 g saturated)
4 g sugar

Even fruit biscuits can contain dangers.

Chocolate

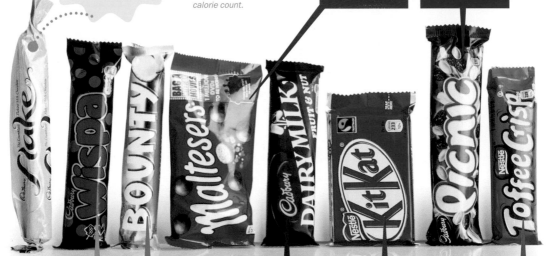

Eat This!

Flake
(1 package, 32 g)

170 calories
9.9 g fat
(6.1 g saturated)
17.7 g sugar

Flake is the winner in the world of chocolate bars. The perfect balance of indulgence and a reasonable calorie count.

Maltesers
(1 package, 37 g)

187 calories
9.1 g fat
(5.6 saturated)
19.7 g sugar

A bag of these treats is a massive 73 calories less than a Mars, with half the sugar.

Picnic
(1 package, 48 g)

230 calories
10.9 g fat
(5.1 g saturated)
22.9 g sugar

Big and chunky enough to give the Lion bar a run for its money, but with 26 fewer calories.

Wispa
(1 package, 39 g)

215 calories
13.1 g fat
(8.2 g saturated)
20.7 g sugar

All those tiny air bubbles add up to fewer calories for you, making this a smarter treat.

Bounty
(1 bar, 28.5 g)

134 calories
6.8 g fat
(5.6 g saturated)
13.6 g sugar

At first glance very light. Be careful though, nutrition is for a single bar and you get two in a pack. Even if you eat the lot it's better than a Boost.

Dairy Milk Fruit & Nut
(1 package, 49 g)

245 calories
13.3 g fat
(7.4 g saturated)
26.8 g sugar

Chunkier than it's all-chocolate cousin – and just a shade healthier. Not that much, mind.

Kit Kat
(1 package, 48 g)

233 calories
11 g fat
(7 g saturated)
22.8 g sugar

Your goal: Pawn off one of the four sticks in this package. You'll make a friend and drop down to a very reasonable 175 calories.

Toffee Crisp
(1 bar, 44 g)

229 calories
12 g fat
(8 g saturated)
21.2 g sugar

A lighter option mainly due to the fact that it's a bit smaller than most other bars. Still, it's one way to make portion control easy.

Not That!

Snickers
(1 bar, 64.5 g)
296 calories
16.4 g fat
(5.5 g saturated)
26.2 g sugars

There's extra protein from the peanuts, but a Snickers also has more calories than a McDonald's cheeseburger

Lion
(1 bar, 52 g)
256 calories
11.9 g fat
(7.4 g saturated)
27.6 g sugar

Believe it or not, the least calorific on this side of the page. But the roar of the Lion still busts the 250 calorie mark.

Mars
(1 package, 58 g)
260 calories
9.9 g fat
(4.8 g saturated)
34.6 g sugar

Mars does manage to keep the fat levels under control – but makes up for it with extra sugar.

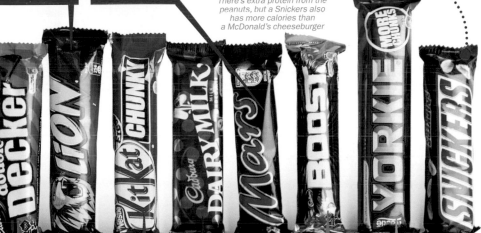

Double Decker
(1 bar, 60 g)
275 calories
11.1 g fat
(6 g saturated)
32.9 g sugar

True to its name this bar packs in double layers of everything, which could translate to extra layers of fat on you.

Kit Kat Chunky
(1 bar, 48 g)
261 calories
13.4 g fat
(7.6 g saturated)
25.1 g sugar

The chunky version of the Kit Kat could make you chunkier, especially as it's harder to share than the original.

Dairy Milk
(1 bar, 49 g)
260 calories
14.6 g fat
(9.1 g saturated)
27.8 g sugar

Solid chocolate – less room for anything with real nutritional value (or even any air, for that matter).

Boost
(1 bar, 60.5 g)
305 calories
17.2 g fat
(12.8 g saturated)
29.9 g sugar

Amazing, really, that they managed to pack so much into such a small package...

Yorkie
(1 bar, 64.5 g)
302 calories
17.4 g fat
(10.3 g saturated)
31.3 g sugar

As you might expect from a bar famed for its size, it's also a fat and calorie fest.

203

Crisps

Eat This!

Yorkshire Crisps Natural Sea Salt
(¼ pack)

122 calories
6 g fat
(1.3 g saturated)
0.2 g salt

Natural sea salt, naturally not a bad crisp.

Tyrrells Sea Salt & Cracked Black pepper
(¼ pack)

182 calories
10.2 g fat
(1 g saturated)
0.5 g salt

These aren't your healthiest crisps. But what is surprising is that they're slightly healthier than the vegetable option

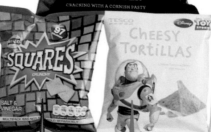

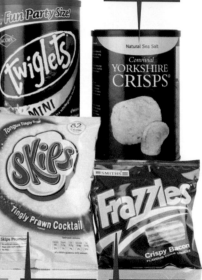

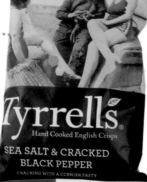

Walkers Quavers
(1 pack)

88 calories
4.9 g fat
(0.4 g saturated)
0.36 g salt

A literally light snack, quavers may be the best of the cheesy crisps.

Walkers Squares
(1 pack)

97 calories
4 g fat
(0.3 g saturated)
0.5 g salt

It may be hip to be square with half the fat content of it's salt and vinegar rival.

Tesco Cheesy Tortillas
(1 pack)

80 calories
1.4 g fat
(0.2 g saturated)
0.3 g salt

Lower in fat than anything on the page, though this is in part due to the small pack.

Jacobs Twiglets
(25 g)

97 calories
3 g fat
(0.4 g saturated)
1.8 g salt

Keep your eye on that salt intake and Twiglets are a welcome edition to the party mix.

KP Skips
(1 pack)

88 calories
4.6 g fat
(0.4 g saturated)
0.4 g salt

Each bag weighs just 17 g, but it's the low calories that count it as a light snack.

Smith's Frazzles
(1 pack)

112 calories
5.3 g fat
(0.5 g saturated)
0.66 g salt

A slightly better option than the Bacon Fries, but still a little calorific.

Yorkshire Crisps Sweet Chilli & Lime

(¼ pack)

130 calories
6 g fat
(1.3 g saturated)
0.55 g salt

Extra seasoning that nudges up calories.

You'd be forgiven for thinking vegetable crisps are healthier. This pack proves that's not always the case.

Not That!

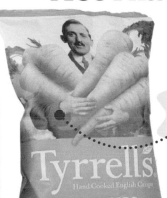

Tyrell's Veg crisps

(¼ pack)

190 calories
12.6 g fat
(1.6 g saturated)
0.25 g salt

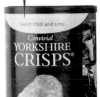

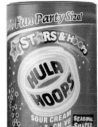

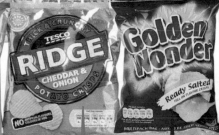

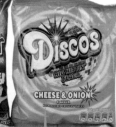

Smith's Bacon Fries

(1 pack)

131 calories
8.5 g fat
(0.8 g saturated)
0.72 g salt

You'd get less fat in eating two rashers of grilled bacon. Might taste better, too.

Walkers Prawn Cocktail

(1 pack)

133 calories
8.2 g fat
(0.6 g saturated)
0.35 g salt

Certainly no fishy goodness contained in these crisps.

KP Sour Cream & Chive Hula Hoops

(25 g)

130 calories
7.2 g fat
(0.7 g saturated)
2 g salt

Starchy Hula Hoops will add to any dieter's woes.

Tesco Ridge Cheese & Oinion

(1 pack)

160 calories
8.8 g fat
(0.9 g saturated)
0.3 g salt

The mighty ridge almost beats all with its calorie count.

Golden Wonder

(1 pack)

131 calories
8.1 g fat
(1 g saturated)
0.5 g salt

No nutritional wonder here, just a crisp with high numbers in all the wrong categories.

Discos Salt & Vinegar

(1 pack)

146 calories
8.3 g fat
(1.6 g saturated)
0.6 g salt

Disco away from these towards a healthier crisp option.

205

Desserts

A better biscuit than most
and now a better cake bar
than others as well.

Jaffa Cake Bar
(1 bar)

94 calories
3.5 g fat
(1.8 g saturated)
11.6 g sugar

Sainsbury's Topsy Turvy Trifle Sundae
(100 g)

216 calories
11.5 g fat
(6.7 g saturated)
17 g sugar

Considering the ingredients the calorie cost has been kept affordable.

Strawberry Cheesecake

Whole juicy strawberries on a deep layer of delicious cheesecake and a crunchy biscuit base.

485 g

McVitie's Jaffa Cakes
5 Cake Bars

94

NEW

Mr KIPLING 2 Exceedingly Good... Puddings
Sticky Toffee
...sponge puddings covered in yummy toffee sauce

Mr KIPLING 6 Exceedingly Good... Country SLICES
...baked with sultanas and currants

Nestlé Aero Bubbly Dessert

Sainsbury's be good to yourself
fresh custard

Mr Kipling Country Slices
(1 cake)

117 calories
5 g fat
(2 g saturated)
13 g sugar

The lightest option available from the kitchen of Mr Kipling.

Conditorei Coppenrath & Wiese Strawberry Cheesecake
(⅙, 81 g)

202 calories
9.9 g fat
(4.9 g saturated)
14.2 g sugar

Just make sure you stick to that sixth.

Mr Kipling Sticky Toffee Sponge Pudding
(1 pudding, 85 g)

266 calories
7.1 g fat
(2.8 g saturated)
33 g sugar

Portion control is the key here. It may be a smaller pot, but that's the sensible option.

Aero Chocolate Mousse
(1 pot, 59 g)

98 calories
3.6 g fat
(2.4 g saturated)
12.9 g sugar

Not just pumped full of it's trademark bubbles. This mousse weighs more for fewer calories. Genius.

Sainsbury's Be Good To Youself Custard
(100 g)

64 calories
1.5 g fat
(1 g saturated)
3.5 g sugar

Good luck finding better. A lean custard that will give you your just desserts.

Not That!

Sainsbury's Rocky Road Sundae
(100 g)

321 calories
19.2 g fat
(11.8 g saturated)
22.8 g sugar

How many layers of chocolate can you see? That's right, too many.

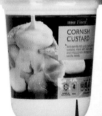

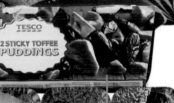

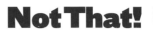

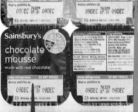

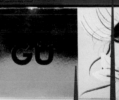

Way more calories than the lighter Jaffa Cake version.

Galaxy Cake Bar
(1 bar)

154 calories
8.8 g fat
(4.4 g saturated)
13.7 g sugar

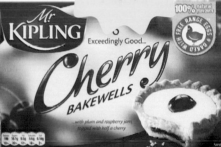

Tesco Finest Cornish Custard
(100 g)

230 calories
16.6 g fat
(10 g saturated)
12.9 g sugar

Not sure how the Cornish like their custard but this triples the calories of its rival.

Sainsbury's Chocolate Mousse
(1 pot, 55 g)

124 calories
8.5 g fat
(5.5 g saturated)
25 g sugar

Twice the fat, sat and sugars of the Aero will have twice the impact on your waistline.

Tesco Sticky Toffee Pudding
(1 pudding, 130 g)

425 calories
20 g fat
(12 g saturated)
48 g sugar

Sticky. Toffee. Pudding. Be prepared for the 48 grams of sugar now.

Gü Chocolate & Vanilla Cheesecake
(1 pot, 90 g)

379 calories
27.1 g fat
(15.9 g saturated)
21.2 g sugar

Luxurious, yes. Healthy, no.

Mr Kipling Cherry Bakewell
(1 cake)

198 calories
9 g fat
(7.8 g saturated)
18 g sugar

With half your RDA saturated fat in one cake this dessert doesn't need the cherry on top.

207

Soft Drinks

Drink This!

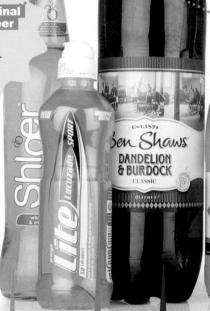
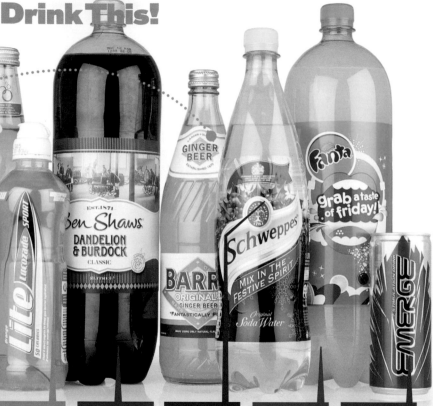

That's a 17.5 calorie saving in a 250ml glass or 70 per litre, over the Jamaican variety, which all adds up.

Schloer White Grape & Elderflower	Lucozade Sport Orange Lite	Ben Shaw Dandelion & Burdock	Schweppes Soda Water	Fanta	Emerge
(100 ml)	(100 ml)	(100 ml)	(100 mL)	(100 mL)	(100 ml)
37 calories 9.2 g sugar	10 calories 1 g sugar	28 calories 6.9 g sugar	0 calories 0 sugar	30 calories 7.1 g sugar	42 calories 9.8 g sugar
Elderflower dilutes that sugary grape juice to a more suitable level.	Ditch the fizzy stuff, grab the lite option and you have just a single gram of sugar to concern yourself.	Yes they still make it, and while the flavour may not be for everyone it is one of the better soft drinks for you.	Just water with added fizz, drink as much of this as you like. Better still add some vodka and lime.	Part of the Coca-Cola corp. yet made to a less sugary recipe, this sweet orange fizz goes low at just 30 cals per 100 mls.	Save yourself a few calories and a gram of sugar by switching over to Emerge.

208

SUPERMARKET TREATS & DRINKS

Not That!

Old Jamacia Ginger Ale
(100 ml)
64 calories
14.1 g sugars

A few more calories and a large bottle to hinder portion control.

Red Bull
(100 ml)
45 calories
11 g sugar

The king of energy drinks has a long list of ingredients meant to give you a boost. Either way that sugar should be of concern.

Irn Bru
(100 ml)
43 calories
10.5 g sugar

Apologies to the Scots, but Irn Bru runs neck and neck with Coke and Red Bull for excessive sugars content.

Schweppes Indian Tonic Water
(100 ml)
37 calories
9 g sugar

That's a lot of sugar for "water" and 37 calories that you wouldn't find normally in H₂O.

Coca Cola
(100 ml)
42 calories
10.6 g sugar

The granddaddy of all fizzy drinks sits unapologetically exactly where you expect it to be. Firmly on the fattening side of the line.

Lucozade Energy Orange
(100 ml)
70 calories
13.8 g sugar

Whether or not it gives you an energy boost, that sugar content may set you up for a crash.

Schloer White Grape
(100 ml)
42 calories
10.4 g sugar

White grapes are one of the most fructose heavy fruits so avoid this 100 percent grape fizz.

209

Ice Cream

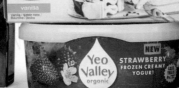

Eat This!

Wall's Viennetta
(100 ml)

120 calories
8 g fat
(7 g saturated)
10 g sugar

Sainsbury's Triple Chocolate
(100 g)

163 calories
7.4 g fat
(4.7 g saturated)
16.8 g sugar

Not just chocolate, but triple chocolate. How much more cocoa do you need? And it still keeps the calories lower than the monkey version.

It's a classic and as ice cream goes, you'll struggle to find anything lower in calories.

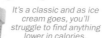

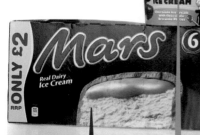

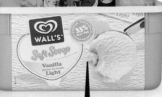

Mars
(1 bar, 51g)

143 calories
8.3 g fat
(5.5 g saturated)
12.1 sugar

Okay, so a Mars a day probably isn't the best idea, but this ice cream bar does nudge it noticably lower in calories and fat compared to its peanut heavy cousin.

Ben & Jerry's Chocolate Fudge Brownie
(100 ml)

210 calories
10 g fat
(7 g saturated)
21 g sugar

This is still very indulgent, but nudges slightly ahead of the Häagen Dazs version in cutting calories and fat.

Yeo Valley Strawberry Frozen Yogurt
(100 ml)

85 calories
1.9 g fat
(1.2 g saturated)
14.3 g sugar

Frozen yogurts wins against ice cream every time, whatever the brand. Fewer calories and a huge cut in fats. Make the switch today.

Wall's Soft Scoop Vanilla
(100 g)

130 calories
6 g fat
(3 g saturated)
17 g sugar

The right way to do vanilla, not just because its easier to scoop and serve, but easy to swallow without so much of a guilty conscience.

Not That!

Sainsbury's Chocolate Monkey Mallow
(100 g)

262 calories
13 g fat
(8.8 g saturated)
28.7 g sugar

What is this monkey business that adds 100 extra calories and 10 grams of sugars to the pot?

Magnum Classic
(1 ice cream)

260 calories
16 g fat
(12 g saturated)
23 g sugar

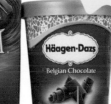

Half you daily amount of saturated fat in a single ice cream? Hmm, maybe look for those mini-Magnums.

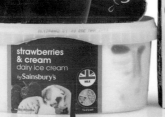

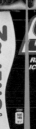

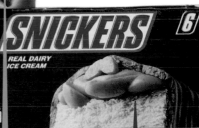

Sainsbry's Taste the Difference Vanilla
(100 g)

242 calories
16.4 g fat
(11.2 g saturated)
17.5 g sugar

Beware: a really creamy vanilla ice cream can ram in more of the big four than a serving of chocolate brownie version.

Sainsbury's Strawberries & Cream
(100 g)

176 calories
7.4 g fat
(4.8 g saturated)
18 g sugars

Not the biggest nutritional offender on the wrong side of the Eat This Not That law, but it just can't compete against fro-yo.

Häagen Dazs Belgian Chocolate
(100 ml)

286 calories
18.6 g fat

Häagen Dazs win the prize for the most indulgent chocolate ice cream of the lot.

Snickers
(1 bar, 53 g)

185 calories
11.2 g fat
(5.9 g saturated)
13.2 g sugar

Peanuts may be a great source of monounsaturated fats, but don't fool yourself into thinking that it means they'll help to keep you trim.

Juice

Drink This!

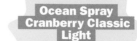

Ocean Spray Cranberry Classic Light
(250 ml)

20 calories
0 g fat
3.5 g sugar

It's light and delicious. And the 25% juice content means it'll still provide a vitamin kick. A clear winner.

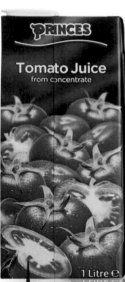

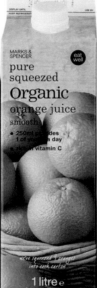

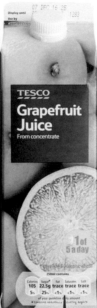

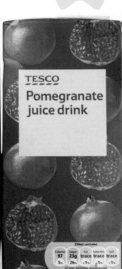

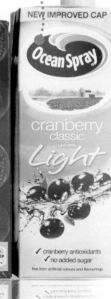

Princes Tomato Juice
(250 ml)

40 calories
0 g fat
8 g sugar

The king of fruit juice. It really doesn't come much healthier than this. The tomatoes will give you a dose of cancer-fighting lycopene, too.

Marks & Spencer Pure Squeezed Orange Juice Smooth
(250 ml)

100 calories
0.3 g fat
23 g sugar

There's only one ingredient in this: oranges (and organic ones at that).

Tesco Grapefruit Juice
(250 ml)

105 calories
0 g fat
22.5 g sugar

Made from concentrate, but all that sugar is natural, plus its antioxidants help boost the body's healing process.

Tesco Pomegranate Juice Drink
(250 mi)

97 calories
0 g fat
23 g sugar

More vitamin C than orange juice, antioxidants that fight cancer. It's so good we'll let it off a bit of extra added sugar.

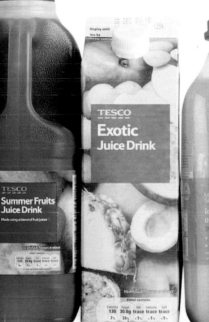

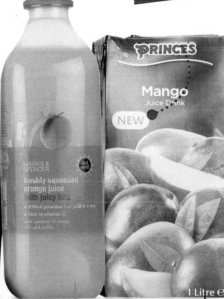

Ocean Spray Cranberry & Raspberry
(250 ml)

120 calories
0 g fat
53 g sugar

Packed full of sugar and only 15% juice – less than the Light version. Not a lot going for it (apart from sugar and water, of course)

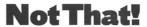

Not That!

NEW & IMPROVED

Ocean Spray

cranberry & raspberry
juice drink

✓100% RDA Vitamin C
free from artificial colours, flavourings and sweeteners

TESCO
Summer Fruits Juice Drink
Made using a blend of fruit juices

Calories	Sugar	Fat	Saturates	Salt
125	29.8g	trace	trace	trace

TESCO
Exotic Juice Drink

Calories	Sugar	Fat	Saturates	Salt
130	30.8g	trace	trace	trace
7%	34%	<1%	<1%	<1%

MARKS & SPENCER
freshly squeezed orange juice with juicy bits
• 230ml provides 1 of your 5 a day
• rich in vitamin C

PRINCES
Mango
Juice Drink
NEW

1 Litre ℮

Tesco Summer Fruits Juice Drink
(250 ml)

125 calories
0 g fat
29.8 g sugar

Basically 30% apple juice concentrate with 1% cherries, 1% strawberries, water, sugar oh, and colouring.

Tesco Exotic Juice Drink
(250 ml)

130 calories
0 g fat
30.8 g sugars

Water and sugar feature highly again here, but to give Tesco their due, there is juice from nine different fruits in this.

Marks & Spencer Freshly Squeezed Orange Juice with Bits
(250 ml)

125 calories
0 g fat
23.3 g sugar

Still 100% oranges but the 'bits' add calories, so opt for a smooth version.

Princes Mango Juice Drink
(250 ml)

135 calories
0 g fat
32 g sugar

As a general rule steer clear of the words 'juice drink' on any brand: they guarantee low fruit content and high sugar.

Snacks

Eat This!

Bundu Original Beef Biltong
(85 g)

204 calories
4.4 g fat
(1.9 g saturated)
2.75 g salt

Similar to jerky, but originating in South Africa, biltong has a less sweet taste and keeps the sat-fat lower.

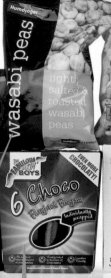
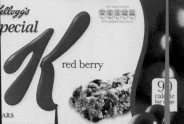
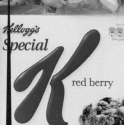
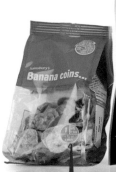
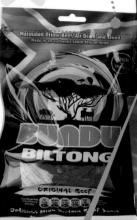

Sainsbury's Banana Coins	Humdinger Wasabi Peas	Fabulous Bakin' Boys Chocolate Oaty Flapjack Fingers	Sainsbury's Japanese Style Rice Crackers	Kellogg's Special K Red Berry cereal bar	Sainsbury's Unsalted Jumbo Peanuts & Raisins
(¼ pack, 25 g)	(100 g)	(1 snack)	(100 g)	(1 bar, 23 g)	(50 g)
88 calories	404 calories	130 calories	387 calories	88 calories	210 calories
0.3 g fat	12 g fat	6.2 g fat	4.6 g fat	1 g fat	10.2 g fat
(0.1 g saturated)	(5 g saturated)	(3.4 g saturated)	(1 g saturated)	(0.8 g saturated)	(1.7 g saturated)
19.2 g sugar	0.9 g salt	9 g sugars	1.45 g salt	9 g sugar	trace salt
Heavy on the sugars, but that's natural from the bananas. A fine fruit treat.	The Japanese outdo the Indians in the snack stakes. You'll save over 100 calories.	Not bad, but just one at a time now.	Beats Branston crackers hands down.	It's a dieter's staple for a reason.	A good trail mix.

Not That!

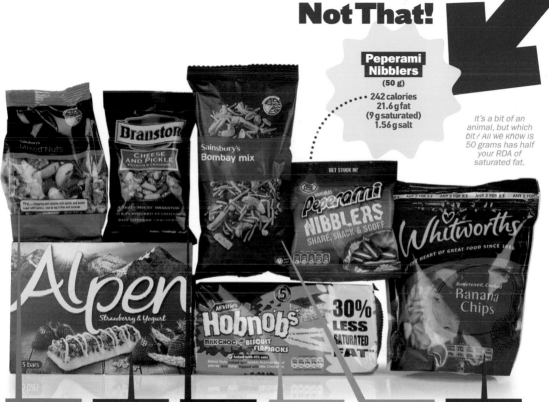

Peperami Nibblers
(50 g)
- 242 calories
- 21.6 g fat
- (9 g saturated)
- 1.56 g salt

It's a bit of an animal, but which bit? All we know is 50 grams has half your RDA of saturated fat.

Sainsbury's Mixed nuts
(50 g)

336 calories
32.4 g fat
(5.3 g saturated,)
trace salt

A really healthy bag of nuts. But from a weight loss point of view, go for a lighter option.

Alpen Strawberry & Yogurt
(1 bar, 29 g)

121 calories
3.1 g fat
(1.8 g saturated)
10.3 g sugar

That yogurt coating worsens the nutrition in this bar.

Branston Peanuts & Crackers
(100 g)

524 calories
34.6 g fat
(3.8 g saturated)
3.8 g salt

A few handfuls could see you with 150 extra calories over rice crackers.

McVities Chocolate Hobnob Flapjack
(1 snack)

152 calories
6 g fat
(2.2 g saturated)
12.5 g sugars

An unhealthy biscuit, makes unhealthy flapjack.

Sainsbury's Bombay Mix
(100 g)

533 calories
33.2 g fat
(5.1 g saturated)
1.68 g salt

A meal's worth of calories from 100 grams? Avoid bowls of these at a party.

Whitworths Banana Chips
(25 g)

130 calories
7.8 g fat
(7.5 g saturated)
5.6 g sugars

Only 55 percent banana, the rest is coconut oil, sugar and flavourings.

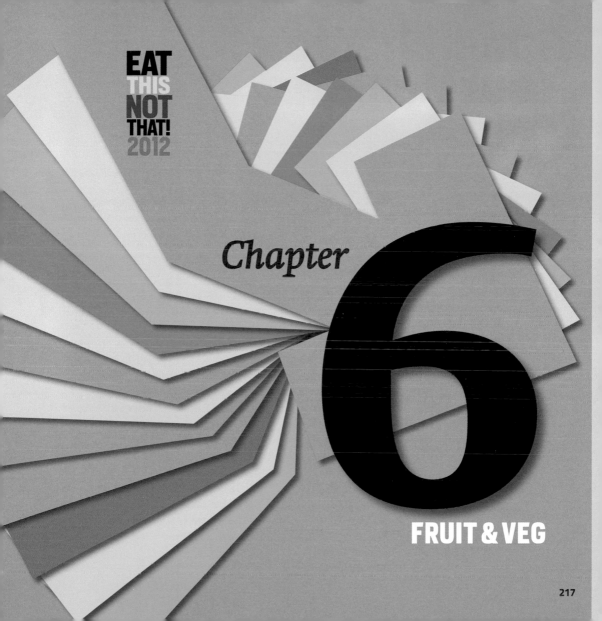

Chapter

6

FRUIT & VEG

Supercharge Your Meals

There's an old joke: a British mother tells her child, "Eat your broccoli. In China, children don't even have broccoli!" Meanwhile, in China, a woman tells her child, "Eat your rice. In Britain, children have to eat broccoli!"

Such is the stigma that we attach to vegetables and, to a lesser extent, to fruit. Eating them is an unpleasant chore, a duty—something we do when we aren't having the fun experience of chilli-drenched nachos and cheese. And that's why the average child in the UK just isn't getting their recommended five-a-day.

In fact, The National Diet and Nutrition Surveys for 2008/09 and 2009/10 showed that 11- to 18-year-old girls consume, on average, only 2.7 of the recommended portions, with just 5 percent consuming what the official guidelines state are needed for good health. Boys of the same age fared little better, with an average of 3.1 portions a day, and just 13 percent having the full five-a-day. And that's with nagging parents looking over the kids' shoulders. What happens when the children grow up and become... us?

Well, it doesn't get any better. Only 29 percent of women and just 20 percent of men consume the recommended amount of produce each day. Which is bad news when you consider that a Harvard study of 110,000 men and women found that those who ate eight or more servings of fruit and vegetables a day were 30 percent less likely to have a heart attack or stroke than those who ate less than 1½ servings a day. You don't have to move into Mr McGregor's garden to reap the health benefits of the veg aisle—indeed, eating just five servings of fruit and vegetables can lower your risk of coronary heart disease and stroke by 20 percent, versus those who eat three or fewer servings per day.

Now, we know what you're thinking. Five servings a day? Eight servings a day? That's a lot of kohlrabi, mate!

But it's not. Here's how you get eight servings without breaking a sweat: have a banana with cereal and a glass of 100 percent fruit juice for breakfast. A side salad at lunch with your sandwich and a piece of fruit. Snack on some raisins when your energy is running low around 3pm. At dinner, have another salad or a vegetable soup and a side of broccoli with your meat. Bang, you're already at seven servings. Chomp on a couple of carrot sticks or have a glass of Innocent Fruit smoothie somewhere in your day and you've done it—how painless was that? And just look at the benefits.

- **You'll lower your blood pressure.** One study found that people with high blood pressure who ate a diet rich in fruit, vegetables and low-fat dairy products reduced their systolic blood pressure by 11 points and their diastolic blood pressure by six points—as much as medications can achieve.

- **You'll protect your eyes.** A University study found that sweet corn, orange bell peppers, kiwi, grapes, spinach, oranges and various squash and leafy green vegetables were packed with the nutrients lutein and zeaxanthin, which have been shown to protect the eyes from macular degeneration.

Trick Your Kids into Loving Vegetables

SHAPE 'EM. A carrot is still a carrot—unless it's shaped like a ninja throwing star! A few quick turns of the knife can make vegetables into cool new edible toys. And don't forget the old trick of spelling out words with green beans.

HIDE 'EM. Throw broccoli, spinach and other veggies into the blender, then spoon them into spaghetti sauce. Blended finely, they become almost invisible, but will still impart their magical nutritional content.

FRENCH FRY 'EM. Even children who hate vegetables love chips. But traditional chips are laden with grease and low in nutrition. Trick your youngsters with baked chips made from thinly cut potatoes, sweet potatoes, carrots and parsnips. Splash them with a little olive oil and paprika and bake at 220°C/gas mark 7 for 30 to 40 minutes.

- **You'll build a leaner body.** Calcium (from kale, broccoli and spinach), potassium (from Swiss chard, lima beans, yams, winter squash and avocado) and magnesium (from potatoes, beans and black-eyed peas) are just three of the essential muscle-building nutrients you can get from vegetables. And the fibre that's packed into most produce will help keep you fuller, longer—which means you'll stay slimmer, longer.

- **You'll have fewer sick days.** The essential antioxidant vitamins— E (from almonds, spinach, broccoli, and peanuts), C (from broccoli, peppers, papaya and kale) and A (from carrots, melon and apricots)—will protect you against everything from wrinkles to heart disease.

Does that get you fired up to dive into the fruit and veg section? It should. The UK's Food Standards Agency says most of us need to increase our consumption of all of the vitamins, minerals and other nutrients above. And eating as many vegetables and fruits as we can get our hands on is the best way to do it. Start today.

Lean, Green Machines

Essentially, iceberg lettuce is the nutritional equivalent of a plastic office plant; it adds a little colour, but mostly it just takes up space. Iceberg may be cheap and plentiful, but it contains almost no fibre, vitamins or minerals. If you're going to eat salad, you might as well eat the power salad. Check out this green dream team.

The Cancer Killer
ROMAINE LETTUCE
This celery-flavoured green is one of the best vegetable sources of beta-carotene—712 micrograms per portion. High levels of beta-carotene inhibit the growth of prostate cancer cells by 50 percent.

The Bone Builder
ROCKET
A handful of these mustard-flavoured leaves has 10 percent of the bone-building mineral found in

a glass of whole milk and 100 percent less saturated fat. There's also magnesium, for more protection against osteoporosis.

The Pipe Protector
WATERCRESS
It's a pepper-flavoured filter for your body. Watercress contains chemicals that may prevent cigarette smoke and other airborne pollutants from causing lung cancer.

The Heart Healer
CHICORY
It's slightly bitter, crisp, and has lots of fibre. A portion provides almost 20 percent of your daily folate. People who don't get enough have a 50 percent greater risk of heart disease.

The Brain Booster
MUSTARD GREENS
These spicy, crunchy greens are packed with the amino acid tyrosine. In a recent military study, researchers found that eating a tyrosine-rich meal an hour before taking a test helped soldiers significantly improve both their memories and their concentration.

The Anti-ageing Agent
BOK CHOY
Think of it as a cabbage-flavoured multivitamin. A bowl of bok choy has 23 percent of your daily requirement of vitamin A and a third of your vitamin C, along with three tongue-twisting, cancer-fighting, age-reducing phytochemicals: flavonoids, isothiocyanates and dithiolthione.

The Sight Sharpener
SPINACH
A top source of lutein and zeaxanthin, two powerful antioxidants that protect your vision from the ravages of old age. A study from Tufts University found that frequent spinach eaters had as much as a 43 percent lower risk of age-related macular degeneration.

The Pressure Punisher
KOHLRABI
Kohlrabi tastes like a cross between a cabbage and a turnip. Each serving contains nearly 25 percent of your daily potassium (to help keep a lid on your blood pressure), along with glucosinolate, a phytochemical that may prevent some cancers.

How to Buy the Best Fruit and Veg

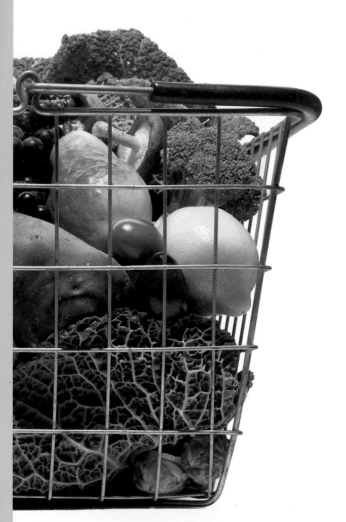

One of the reasons Italians eat so well is that every last one of them believes it is their fundamental right to walk out of the supermarket with the very best ingredients. They won't settle for a wrinkled aubergine, a withered artichoke or an apple that tastes like polystyrene. And neither should you. But the problem is, finding the best, ripest, tastiest fruits and vegetables isn't as intuitive as you might think. It's a task that requires the attention of all five senses in order to pick up on the subtleties and nuances behind ultimate ripeness and utmost quality.

Regardless of what fruit or veg you are shopping for, start with these three basic rules.

1 **Beautiful doesn't mean delicious.** Sub-par conventional produce is bred to look waxy, glistening and perfectly symmetrical, while prime fruits and vegetables are often irregularly shaped, with slight visual imperfections outside but a world of flavour waiting inside.

2 **Use your hands.** You can learn more about a fruit or vegetable from picking it up than you can from staring it down. Heavy, sturdy fruits and vegetables with taut skin and peels are signs of freshness.

3 **Shop with the seasons.** Of course, sometimes you just need a tomato, but there are two great reasons to shop in season: it's cheaper and it's better for you. We asked Aliza Green, author of *Field Guide to Produce* for the inside track on scoring the best of the bounty. Use the tips and tricks that follow and you'll bring home the best fruits and vegetables every time, just like an Italian.

THE FRUIT 'N' VEG DECODER

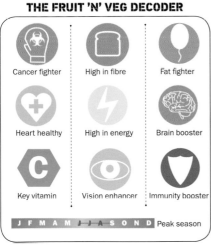

Cancer fighter	High in fibre	Fat fighter
Heart healthy	High in energy	Brain booster
C — Key vitamin	Vision enhancer	Immunity booster

`J F M A M J J A S O N D` Peak season

Apples

PERFECT PICK
Firm and heavy for its size with smooth, matte, unbroken skin and no bruising. The odd blemish or brown "scald" streaks do not negatively impact flavour. The smaller the apple, the bigger the flavour.

PEAK SEASON
`J F M A M J J A S O N D`

HANDLE WITH CARE Keep apples in a plastic bag in the fridge but away from vegetables. Here, they should remain edible for several weeks.

THE PAYOFF Quercetin, a flavonoid linked to better heart health, plus the soluble fibre pectin, which keeps cholesterol in check.

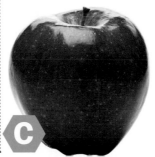

Artichokes

PERFECT PICK
Deep green and heavyset with undamaged, tightly closed leaves. The leaves should squeak when pinched together. One that is starting to open is past its best days.

PEAK SEASON
`J F M A M J J A S O N D`

HANDLE WITH CARE Store in the fridge in a plastic bag for up to 5 days.

THE PAYOFF A higher total antioxidant capacity than any other vegetable.

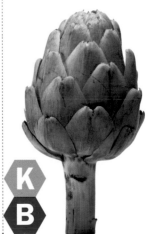

Asparagus

PERFECT PICK
Vibrant green spears with tight purple-tinged buds. Avoid spears that are fading in colour or wilting. Thinner spears are sweeter and more tender.

PEAK SEASON
`J F M A M J J A S O N D`

HANDLE WITH CARE Trim the woody ends and stand upright a little water in a tall container. Cover the tops with a plastic bag and cook within a few days.

THE PAYOFF Folate, a type of B vitamin that can protect the heart by helping to reduce inflammation.

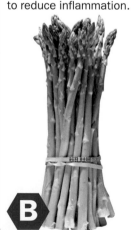

Aubergine

PERFECT PICK
Good weight to them with tight, shiny skin. When they're pressed, look for them to be springy, not spongy. The stem and cap should be forest green, not browning.

PEAK SEASON
`J F M A M J J A S O N D`

HANDLE WITH CARE Store in a cool place (not the fridge). Aubergines are quite sensitive to the cold.

THE PAYOFF Chlorogenic acid, a phenol antioxidant that scavenges disease-causing free radicals.

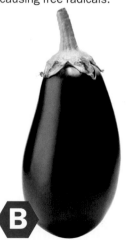

Avocados

PERFECT PICK
Firm to the touch without any sunken, mushy spots. They shouldn't rattle if shaken—a sign the pit has pulled away from the flesh.

PEAK SEASON
`J F M A M J J A S O N D`

HANDLE WITH CARE To ripen, place in a paper bag and store at room temperature. To speed up this process, add an apple to the bag: it emits ripening ethylene gas. Ripe avocados keep for a week in the fridge.

THE PAYOFF Plenty of cholesterol-lowering monounsaturated fat.

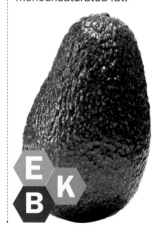

Baby Spinach

PERFECT PICK
Opt for bunches with leaves that are crisp and verdant green, with no spots, yellowing or limpness. Thin stems are best as thick ones are a sign of more bitter, overgrown leaves.

PEAK SEASON

J F M A M J J A S O N D

HANDLE WITH CARE Pack spinach loosely in a plastic bag and store in the fridge for up to four days.

THE PAYOFF Chromium, which is involved in carbohydrate and fat metabolism and may reduce hunger and food intake.

Bananas

PERFECT PICK
Ripe bananas have uniform yellow skins or small brown freckles indicating they are at their sweetest. Avoid any with evident bruising or split skins.

PEAK SEASON

J F M A M J J A S O N D

HANDLE WITH CARE Store unripe bananas on the work top, away from direct heat and sunlight (speed things up by placing green bananas in an open paper bag). Once ripened, refrigerate; though the peel turns brown, the flavour and quality are unaffected.

THE PAYOFF Vitamin B6, which helps prevent cognitive decline.

Beetroot

PERFECT PICK
Smooth, deep-red surface that's unyielding when pressed. Smaller roots are sweeter and more tender. Attached greens should be deep green and not withered.

PEAK SEASON

J F M A M J J A S O N D

HANDLE WITH CARE Remove the leaves (which are great fried in olive oil) and store in a plastic bag in the fridge for no more than two days. The beetroot will last for up to two weeks.

THE PAYOFF Nitrate, which may help lower blood pressure.

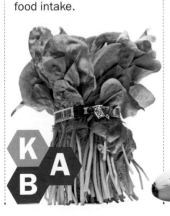

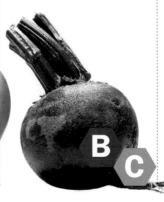

Blueberries

PERFECT PICK

Plump, uniform indigo berries with taut skin and a dull white bloom. Check the bottom of the container for juice stains indicating many crushed berries. Those with a red or green tinge will never fully ripen.

PEAK SEASON

J F M A M J J A S O N D

HANDLE WITH CARE Transfer, unwashed, to an airtight container and refrigerate for five to seven days. Blueberries spoil quickly if left at room temperature.

THE PAYOFF More disease-fighting antioxidants (especially in the wild berries) than most other common fruits.

Broccoli

PERFECT PICK

Rigid stems with tightly formed floret clusters that are deep green or tinged purple. Pass on any with yellowing heads—they will inevitably be more bitter.

PEAK SEASON

J F M A M J J A S O N D

HANDLE WITH CARE Place in a plastic bag and store in the refrigerator for up to a week.

THE PAYOFF Sulforaphane, which activates enzymes that seek out and destroy cancerous cells.

Brussels Sprouts

PERFECT PICK

Compact, tight and unshrivelled heads that are vibrant green and feel overweight for their size. Select ones of similar size for ease of cooking, knowing that smaller sprouts pack sweeter flavour.

PEAK SEASON

J F M A M J J A S O N D

HANDLE WITH CARE Refrigerate, unwashed, in a tightly wrapped perforated plastic bag for up to two weeks.

THE PAYOFF Nitrogen compounds called indoles, which have cancer-protecting efficacy.

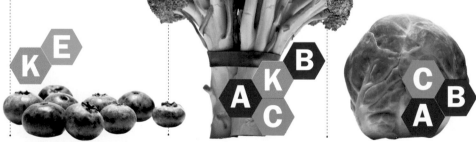

Butternut Squash

PERFECT PICK
Should feel dense for its size with a rind that is smooth, hard, uniformly tan and free of splits. Being able to easily push a fingernail into the rind or scrape bits off indicates an immature, less flavourful squash.

PEAK SEASON
J F M A M J J A S O N D

HANDLE WITH CARE
Butternut should be stored outside the fridge in a cool, well-ventilated, dark place, where it will stay edible for up to three months.

THE PAYOFF Huge amount of vitamin A to ramp up your immune system.

Cabbage

PERFECT PICK
Tightly packed, crisp, deeply hued leaves free of blemishes. Should feel dense when lifted; it's best that the stem not have any cracks at its base.

PEAK SEASON
J F M A M J J A S O N D

HANDLE WITH CARE Tightly enclose cabbage in a plastic bag and store in the fridge for up to 10 days.

THE PAYOFF More than half your vitamin K requirement in just one serving.

Cantaloupe Melon

PERFECT PICK
The stem end should be smooth. Look for a sweet aroma, slightly oval shape, and a good coverage of netting. The blossom end should give slightly to pressure. Avoid those with soft spots—an indication of an over-ripe melon.

PEAK SEASON
J F M A M J J A S O N D

HANDLE WITH CARE Ripe cantaloupes should be stored in the fridge for up to five days, after which they begin to lose flavour.

THE PAYOFF Loads of vitamin C, which may offer protection against having a stroke.

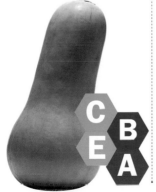

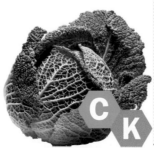

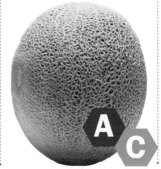

Carrots

PERFECT PICK
Smooth and firm with bright colour. Avoid any that are bendy or cracked. Bright green tops are your freshest choice.

PEAK SEASON

J F M A M J J A S O N D

HANDLE WITH CARE Store in the fridge with the greens removed for three weeks.

THE PAYOFF Beta-carotene, the source of vitamin A, which helps beat infections.

Cauliflower

PERFECT PICK
Ivory white and compact florets with no dark spotting on them or the leaves. The leaves should be verdant and perky.

PEAK SEASON

J F M A M J J A S O N D

HANDLE WITH CARE Refrigerate, unwashed, in a plastic bag for up to a week. If light brown spots develop on the florets, shave off with a paring knife before cooking.

THE PAYOFF Detoxifying compounds called isothiocyanates, which offer protection against aggressive forms of prostate cancer.

Celery

PERFECT PICK
Solid, tight stalks with only a few, if any, cracks and vivid green, not yellowing leaves. The darker the celery, the stronger the flavour.

PEAK SEASON

J F M A M J J A S O N D

HANDLE WITH CARE Store in the fridge for two weeks.

THE PAYOFF Luteolin, a flavonoid linked to reduced brain inflammation, a risk factor for Alzheimer's.

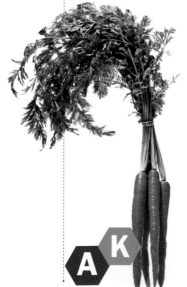

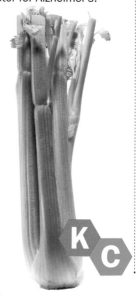

Courgettes

PERFECT PICK

Purchase heavy, tender courgettes with unblemished deep-green skins that are adorned with faint gold specks or strips. The smaller ones are the most flavourful.

PEAK SEASON

J F M A M J J A S O N D

HANDLE WITH CARE
Refrigerate in a plastic bag for up to five days.

THE PAYOFF Riboflavin, a B vitamin needed for red blood cell production and for converting carbohydrates to energy.

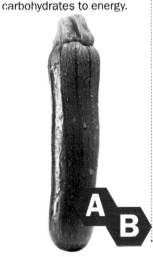

Fennel

PERFECT PICK

Bulbs should be uniform in colour, with no browning and a clean, aroma. Smaller bulbs have a sweeter liquorice-like flavour. Leave bulbs with wilted fronds behind.

PEAK SEASON

J F M A M J J A S O N D

HANDLE WITH CARE
Separate the greens and bulbs and keep each, unwashed, in a plastic bag in the refrigerator for three to five days.

THE PAYOFF Anethole, a phytonutrient that may lessen inflammation and cancer risk.

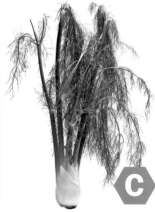

Garlic

PERFECT PICK

The bulb should feel heavy for its size, with tightly closed cloves in the bulb that remain firm when gently pressed. The skin can be pure white or have purple-tinged stripes and should be tight fitting.

PEAK SEASON

J F M A M J J A S O N D

HANDLE WITH CARE Place bulbs in a cool, dark, well-ventilated location for up to a month.

THE PAYOFF The cancer-fighting compound allicin, that can also cut down Helicobacter pylori—bacteria responsible for the development of stomach ulcers.

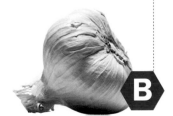

Grapefruit

PERFECT PICK
Opt for a heavy fruit (a sign of juiciness) with thin skin that is a tad responsive to a squeeze. Small imperfections in colour and skin surface are not detrimental to the sweet-tart flavour. Yet, avoid any that are very rough or have soft spots.

PEAK SEASON
J F M A M J J A S O N D

HANDLE WITH CARE
Store refrigerated for two to three weeks.

THE PAYOFF Cancer-preventing lycopene and 120 percent of your vitamin C RDA in just one serving.

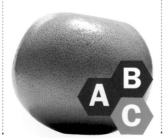

Grapes

PERFECT PICK
Plump, wrinkle-free and firmly attached to the stems. There should be no browning at the stem connection, but a silvery white powder ("bloom") keeps grapes, especially darker ones, fresher longer. Red grapes are best if full-coloured with no green tinge. Green grapes with a yellowish hue are the ripest and sweetest.

PEAK SEASON
J F M A M J J A S O N D

HANDLE WITH CARE
Store, unwashed, in a shallow bowl in the fridge for up to a week.

THE PAYOFF Resveratrol, a potent antioxidant in red/purple grapes that offers protection against cardiovascular disease.

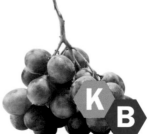

Green Beans

PERFECT PICK
Vibrant, smooth surface without any visible withering. They should "snap" when gently bent.

PEAK SEASON
J F M A M J J A S O N D

HANDLE WITH CARE
Refrigerate, unwashed, in an unsealed bag for up to a week.

THE PAYOFF Their overall antioxidant capacity puts them way ahead of their pea and bean cousins.

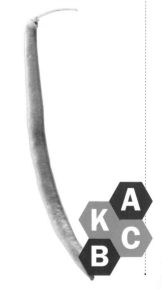

Kale

PERFECT PICK
Dark blue-green colour with moist, jaunty leaves. The smaller the leaves, the more tender the kale. Avoid wilted foliage with discoloured spots.

PEAK SEASON
J F M A M J J A S O N D

HANDLE WITH CARE
Peppery kale is best kept in the fridge wrapped in a plastic bag pierced for aeration, where it will last three to four days.

THE PAYOFF Antioxidant for the retina that protects against vision loss.

Kiwi

PERFECT PICK
A ready-to-devour kiwi will be slightly yielding to the touch. Steer clear of those that are mushy, wrinkled, or bruised with an "off" smell.

PEAK SEASON
J F M A M J J A S O N D

HANDLE WITH CARE Store at room temperature to ripen. To quicken the process, place in a paper bag with an apple. Once ripened, keep in the fridge for up to a week.

THE PAYOFF Only 56 calories for a large one and 20 percent more of the antioxidant vitamin C than an orange.

Leeks

PERFECT PICK
Green, crisp tops with an unblemished white root end. Gravitate toward small- to medium-size leeks, which are less woody and tough than larger ones. Those with spotted or yellowing leaves should be ignored.

PEAK SEASON
J F M A M J J A S O N D

HANDLE WITH CARE Stored loosely wrapped in plastic in the fridge, they'll keep fresh for a week.

THE PAYOFF Good amounts of eye-protecting lutein, manganese.

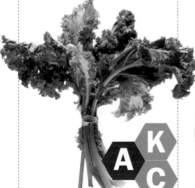

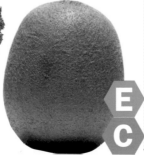

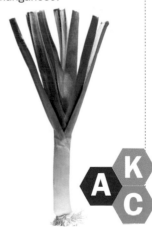

Lemons & limes

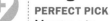

PERFECT PICK
Brightly coloured, well-shaped with smooth, thin skin. They should feel sturdy but give ever so slightly when squeezed. Small brown splotches on limes do not affect flavour (although they are a sign of deterioration). Lemons should have no hint of green.

LEMON PEAK SEASON

J F M A M J J A S O N D

LIME PEAK SEASON

J F M A M J J A S O N D

HANDLE WITH CARE Store at room temperature, in a dark location, for a week or refrigerate for up to two weeks.

THE PAYOFF Phytonutrient liminoids, which appear to have anticancer and antiviral properties.

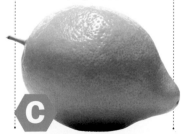

Lettuce: Romaine

PERFECT PICK
The ideal Caesar salad staple has crisp leaves that are free of browning edges and rust spots. The interior leaves are paler in colour with more delicate flavour.

PEAK SEASON

J F M A M J J A S O N D

HANDLE WITH CARE
Refrigerate romaine for up to a week in a plastic bag.

THE PAYOFF Vitamin K, which is needed for blood clotting and bone health.

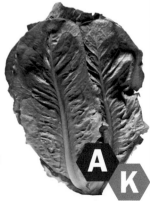

Mangoes

PERFECT PICK
Mangoes to be eaten shortly after purchase should have red skin with splotches of yellow and the soft flesh should give with gentle pressure. Mangoes for later use will be firmer with a tight skin, a duller colour and green near the stem.

PEAK SEASON

J F M A M J J A S O N D

HANDLE WITH CARE Ripen at room temperature until fragrant and giving. Ripe mangoes can be stored in the fridge for up to five days.

THE PAYOFF A good showing of vitamins A, B6 and C, plus fibre.

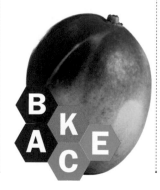

Mushrooms

PERFECT PICK

Tightly closed, firm caps that are not slimy or riddled with dark soft spots. Open caps with visible gills indicate consumption should be a priority.

PEAK SEASON

`J F M A M J J A S O N D`

HANDLE WITH CARE Place meaty mushrooms on a flat surface, cover with a damp paper towel and refrigerate for three to five days.

THE PAYOFF Immune-boosting, tumour-suppressing complex-carbohydrate polysaccharides.

Onions

PERFECT PICK

Nicely shaped with no swelling at the neck and dry, crisp outer skin. Lackluster onions have soft spots, green sprouts or dark patches.

PEAK SEASON

`J F M A M J J A S O N D`

HANDLE WITH CARE Keep onions in a cool, dark location away from potatoes, for around three four weeks.

THE PAYOFF A peptide called GPCS, shown to reduce bone loss in rats, plus the cancer-fighting compound quercetin.

Oranges

PERFECT PICK

Look for the bright, smooth skin then feel for a firm texture. The heavier in the hand, the juicier the orange will be. Avoid any fruit with wrinkled or discoloured skin.

PEAK SEASON

`J F M A M J J A S O N D`

HANDLE WITH CARE Oranges retain their nutritional value for up to two weeks, in or out of the fridge. Keep them unwrapped and dry to avoid mould developing.

THE PAYOFF The hesperidin, a flavanone in oranges has been shown to lower blood pressure and cholesterol. But it's the vitamin C content that makes oranges essential – one will provide your entire RDA.

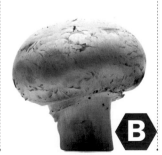

B

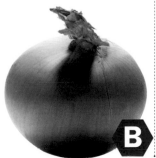

B

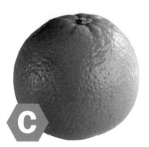

C

Papayas

PERFECT PICK
Beginning to turn yellow with yielding flesh when lightly squeezed. Avoid papayas that are very green, have dark spots or are shrivelled. Blotchy papayas can have the most flavour.

PEAK SEASON
J F M A M J J A S O N D

HANDLE WITH CARE Once ripe, eat or refrigerate for up to three days. Unripe papayas should be ripened at room temperature in a dark place until yellow blotches start to appear.

THE PAYOFF An all-rounder that includes plenty of fibre and vitamins.

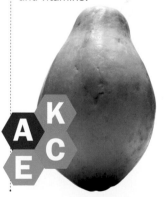

Peaches

PERFECT PICK
Fruity aroma with a background colour of yellow or warm cream. Those destined for immediate consumption yield to gentle pressure along their seams without being too soft. For future intake, opt for those that are firm but not rock hard. Red blush on their cheeks is variety dependent and is not a ripeness indicator.

PEAK SEASON
J F M A M J J A S O N D

HANDLE WITH CARE Store unripe peaches at room temperature open to air. Once ripe, keep in the refrigerator and consume within three days.

THE PAYOFF Vitamin C, antioxidant beta-carotene, fibre and potassium.

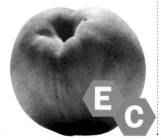

Pears

PERFECT PICK
Pleasant fragrance with some softness at the stem end. The skin should be free of bruises, but some brown discolouration is fine. Firmer pears are preferable for cooking use.

PEAK SEASON
J F M A M J J A S O N D

HANDLE WITH CARE Ripen at room temperature in a loosely closed brown paper bag. Refrigerate once they're ripe and consume within a couple days.

THE PAYOFF Belly-busting fibre and vitamin C—if you eat them with the skin on.

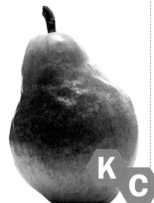

Peppers

PERFECT PICK
Lots of heft for their size with a brightly coloured, wrinkle-free exterior. The stems should be a lively green.

PEAK SEASON

J F M A M J **J A S O N D**

HANDLE WITH CARE Keep in your fridge's veg drawer for up to two weeks.

THE PAYOFF All bell peppers are loaded with antioxidants, especially vitamin C. Red peppers lead the pack, with nearly three times the amount of vitamin C found in fresh oranges. A single serving also has a full day's worth of vision-protecting vitamin A.

Pineapple

PERFECT PICK
Look for vibrant green leaves with a bit of softness and a sweet fragrant aroma from the stem end. Avoid spongy fruit with brown leaves and/or a fermented odour.

PEAK SEASON

J F M A M J J A S O N D

HANDLE WITH CARE Keep a hard pineapple at room temperature for three days until it softens slightly. Then refrigerate for up to five days.

THE PAYOFF Bromelain, compounds with potent anti-inflammatory powers.

Pomegranates

PERFECT PICK
Go for fruits that are weighty for their size with glossy, taut, uncracked skin that is deep red. Gently press the crown end—if a powdery cloud emanates, then the fruit is past its prime.

PEAK SEASON

J F M A M J **J A S O N D**

HANDLE WITH CARE Stored in a cool, dry location, pomegranates keep fresh for several weeks (up to two months in the fridge).

THE PAYOFF Hefty amounts of antioxidants are shown to improve sperm quality, thus boosting fertility, as well as bolstering your immune system.

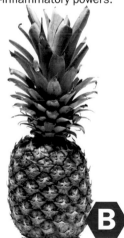

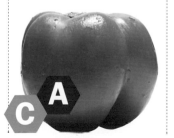

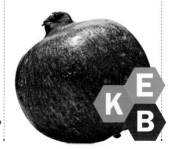

Potatoes: Sweet, White

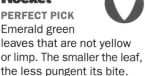

PERFECT PICK
Unyielding, with smooth undamaged skin. Avoid if bruised, cracked or green tinged. Loose spuds tend to be better quality than bagged ones.

PEAK SEASON, SWEET

J F M A M J J A **S O N D**

PEAK SEASON, WHITE

J **F M A M J J A S O N D**

HANDLE WITH CARE
Outside of the fridge, in a cool, dark place (separate from onions), potatoes will last for months. Sweet potatoes, however, should be used within a week.

THE PAYOFF Potassium, which may help preserve muscle mass as we age.

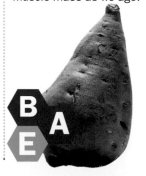

Raspberries

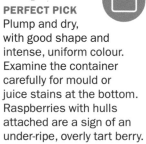

PERFECT PICK
Plump and dry, with good shape and intense, uniform colour. Examine the container carefully for mould or juice stains at the bottom. Raspberries with hulls attached are a sign of an under-ripe, overly tart berry.

PEAK SEASON

J F M A **M J J A S O N D**

HANDLE WITH CARE
Place highly perishable raspberries, unwashed, on a paper towel in a single layer. Cover with a damp paper towel and refrigerate for no more than three days.

THE PAYOFF More fibre (8g per serving) than any other commonly consumed berry. Plus, the anticancer chemical ellagic acid.

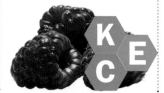

Rocket

PERFECT PICK
Emerald green leaves that are not yellow or limp. The smaller the leaf, the less pungent its bite.

PEAK SEASON

J F **M A M J J A S O N D**

HANDLE WITH CARE
Enclose roots in a damp paper towel and place the leaves in a plastic bag. Store in the fridge for two to three days.

THE PAYOFF Vitamin K, which may improve insulin sensitivity, offering protection against diabetes.

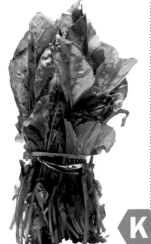

Strawberries
PERFECT PICK
Seek out unblemished berries where the bright red colour extends all the way to the stem. Good berries should have a strong fruity smell and be neither soft and mushy nor hard and firm. Smaller strawberries often have more flavour than the oversized supermarket versions.

PEAK SEASON
J F M A M J J A S O N D

HANDLE WITH CARE Place unwashed strawberries in a single layer on a paper towel in a covered container. They will last for around two to three days in the fridge.

THE PAYOFF The most vitamin C of any of the commonly consumed summer berries.

Tomatoes
PERFECT PICK
Go only for heavy tomatoes that are rich in colour and free of wrinkles, cracks, bruises or spots. They should have some give, unlike the rock-solid ones bred for transport. Too soft, though, and the tomato is over-ripe and watery. Off-season, select more flavourful smaller versions such as Roma and cherry tomatoes.

PEAK SEASON
J F M A M J J A S O N D

HANDLE WITH CARE Never store tomatoes in the fridge; the cool temperatures destroy flavour and texture. Keep them out of direct sunlight for up to a week.

THE PAYOFF Lycopene, a carotenoid antioxidant that helps fend off prostate cancer.

Watermelon
PERFECT PICK
Symmetrical, dense melons that are free of cuts and sunken areas. The rind should appear dull, not shiny, with a rounded creamy-yellow underside that shows where ground ripening took place. A slap should produce a hollow thump.

PEAK SEASON
J F M A M J J A S O N D

HANDLE WITH CARE Store whole in the fridge for up to a week. The cold prevents the flesh from drying out and turning fibrous.

THE PAYOFF Citrulline, an amino acid that's converted to arginine, which relaxes blood vessels, thus improving blood flow.

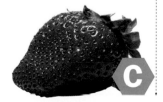
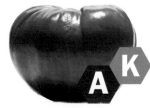
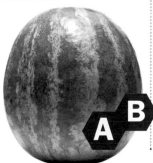

237

FlavourSavers

DITCH THE SALT AND BOOST FLAVOURS THE HEALTHY WAY

ROSEMARY

THE BENEFIT Call it the smart herb. Many people swear by rosemary's ability to increase cognitive functioning, and researchers in California have identified carnosic acid as an active ingredient in rosemary that can offset cognitive degeneration, protect against Alzheimer's and prevent stroke.

THE BLUEPRINT *Mix together minced rosemary, garlic, lemon juice and olive oil. Use as a marinade for chicken, steak, pork, and vegetables.*

BASIL

THE BENEFIT Basil is rich in carotenoids, a class of potent antioxidants that mop up cell-damaging free radicals inside the body. This can help prevent a host of unwanted conditions, such as osteoporosis, arthritis and high cholesterol. Basil also contains oils that prevent bacteria growth and inflammation.

THE BLUEPRINT *Make fresh pesto by blending 2 handfuls fresh basil leaves with 2 tablespoons pine nuts, 22g Parmesan and 60ml olive oil.*

PEPPERMINT

THE BENEFIT Thank the menthol in peppermint for the plant's ability to clear phlegm and mucus from the bronchial tract to facilitate easy breathing. And also for soothing indigestion, gas, menstrual cramps and irritable bowel syndrome.

THE BLUEPRINT *Brighten up a batch of fruit salad with a squeeze of lime and a handful of chopped mint leaves.*

SAGE

THE BENEFIT Like rosemary, sage is known to strengthen memory. The rosemerinic acid in these plants also works to preserve your body by protecting your cells from oxidative damage and alleviating the effects of asthma and arthritis.

THE BLUEPRINT *For a quick pasta sauce, melt a knob of butter in a pan, then add a handful of whole sage leaves. Toss with shop-bought cheese or pumpkin ravioli.*

THYME
THE BENEFIT This tiny herb is extremely rich in iron, which is crucial to your body's ability to transport oxygen. Just 2 teaspoons contain 20 percent of your daily intake. Plus, seasoning with thyme helps protect food from bacterial contamination.

THE BLUEPRINT *Thyme is the ultimate utility player; it goes well with roasted meat and vegetables, tomato sauce, and scrambled eggs.*

CORIANDER
THE BENEFIT Studies on mice found that coriander seeds encouraged the pancreas to produce more insulin—the hormone that helps shuttle glucose into the cells to be burned as energy. This prevents excess blood sugars from being stored as fat. Coriander leaves have the same benefits.

THE BLUEPRINT *Chop up a few tomatoes, an onion and a jalapeño and mix with a heap of coriander for a versatile, fresh salsa.*

PARSLEY
THE BENEFIT These dainty leaves are highly concentrated with luteolin, a powerful flavonoid with anti-inflammatory properties. Researchers at the University of Illinois found that luteolin decreased inflammation in the brain, which helps prevent decline in cognitive functions.

THE BLUEPRINT *Chop and mix it with bulgur wheat. Add olive oil, lemon juice, and mint and you have a tasty tabbouleh salad to pair with grilled fish or meat.*

TARRAGON
THE BENEFIT By increasing the secretion of bile and acids into the stomach, tarragon improves gastric efficiency and whets the appetite. Because of this, it's best used early in the meal as a starter.

THE BLUEPRINT *Grill a mixture of vegetables—onions, peppers, squash, asparagus—and sprinkle them with fresh goat cheese, tarragon, lemon juice and olive oil.*

OREGANO
THE BENEFIT A USDA study found that when adjusted for weight, it had four times the antioxidant activity of blueberries. That means big cancer-fighting potential for your next pizza or pasta sauce.

THE BLUEPRINT *Add equal parts fresh parsley and oregano to a blender and, with the motor running, slowly drizzle in olive or canola oil. Strain and use the infused oil to top grilled fish or chicken, or as a dip for toasted bread.*

The Top 10 Herbs & Spices

So how do you know how to stock the healthiest larder? Italian researchers tested several popular herbs and spices for their content of disease-fighting antioxidants and then ranked them. Although little-used saffron and bay leaf top the list, the scientists found that you can hardly do better than good ol' black pepper. Here's their top 10:

Antioxidant capacity (millimoles per kilogram)

1. Saffron: 53
2. Bay Leaf: 47.9
3. Rosemary: 44
4. Paprika: 40
5. Black Pepper: 37
6. Oregano: 30.7
7. Thyme: 30.5
8. Sage: 23.4
9. Basil: 21.8
10. Mint: 8.8

239

The Organic Decoder

THE FIVE MOST IMPORTANT QUESTIONS ABOUT ORGANIC FOOD ANSWERED

IS ORGANIC WORTH THE EXTRA COST?

The short answer is yes, but it's a little bit more complicated than that. As anyone who's been to a farmers' market can tell you, organic products cost quite a bit more—according to a 2006 study in the *Journal of Food Science,* an average of 10 percent to 40 percent more for typical food items. And while a thinner wallet should be seen as a small price to pay for protecting yourself from pesticides and fertilisers, some organic food is almost nutritionally identical to its conventional counterpart. Take, for example, the humble onion: according to an extensive analysis by the Environmental Working Group, it's got the lowest pesticide load of all the 45 fruits and vegetables that were tested. Also on the produce honour roll are avocados and asparagus. Really torn on whether or not to spend your hard-earned cash on organic? To see how your favourite fruit fares under the pressures of industrial agriculture, check out the table to the right.

IS ORGANIC BETTER FOR ME?

Yes and no. For every study that says organic food has higher concentrations of nutrients, there's another one that denies it. Researchers at the University of California at Davis found that organic kiwis had substantially more disease-fighting polyphenols than conventionally grown kiwis. The problem is, the same team of researchers found the opposite to be true of organic tomatoes—that organically grown tomatoes may have lower levels of antioxidants.

IS ORGANIC BETTER FOR THE EARTH?

In many respects, this may be the biggest reason to go organic. In fact, the certification criteria of the Soil Association specifically says that organic food must be produced using

Should you buy organic fruit and vegetables?

Sometimes the trip to the farmers' market is worth it. That's because buying organic produce can help you avoid pesticides, which may be more prevalent than you think. Friends of the Earth recently tested common fruits and vegetables in the UK to assess the amount of pesticide residue left on them. Here we compile the key findings. The number below each food indicates the percentage of food tested that had the chemical residue. A high figure means you should ditch the regular sort and go organic.

Oranges
98

Almost every non-organic orange will have pesticide residue.

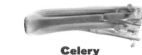

Celery
70

Healthy it may be, but pesticide free? Not so much.

Strawberries
70

The summer treat ranks high on the list of offenders.

Pesticide levels in regular versions high, so buy organic

Pear
66

Non-organic pears have a 66 percent chance of contamination.

Apple
49

Nearly half of all non-organic apples have pesticide residue.

Peach
43

Improving odds, but good enough?

Pesticide levels in regular versions high, so buy organic

Tomato
21

Low levels of chemicals means non-organic is still a good buy.

Mushroom
16

Coming out of the dirt, mushrooms come up respectably clean.

Cauliflower
0

Clean and clear, regular cauliflowers are as good as organic.

Pesticide levels already low, so no need to buy organic

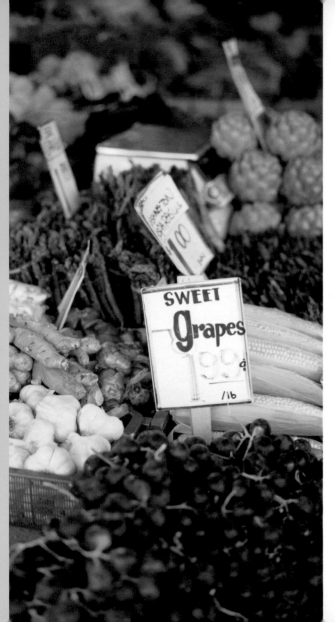

environmentally and animal friendly farming methods on organic farms. This goes beyond cutting out pesticides and fertilisers that can be harmful to people and animals; it involves methods that actually improve the soil—this means using cover crops, manure and crop rotations to fertilise; grazing animals on mixed forage pastures; using renewable resources; and conserving both soil and also water.

But there are two sides to that coin. Researchers at the University of Alberta found that the environmental cost of greenhouse gas emitted to transport organically grown produce was usually comparable to the environmental cost to transport conventional fruit and vegetables. Your best bet: head to the farmers' market. While smaller farms don't always have the means to obtain official organic certification, you'll often find, after chatting with the farmers, that they use sustainable, healthy, environmentally friendly growing and transporting methods that are as good for the planet as they are for your palate.

ARE ORGANIC PACKAGED FOODS BETTER FOR ME?

When it comes to packaged and processed foods, "organic" does not equal "healthy." As Michael Pollan quips in his "eater's manifesto," *In Defense of Food,* Organic chocolate biscuits are not a health food – they're still a heavily processed treat filled with fat and sugar, and your body metabolises organic fat and sugar the same way it does conventional.

DOES ORGANIC TASTE BETTER?

This is perhaps the most important question for discerning cooks the world over. Most chefs and organic enthusiasts would undoubtedly say so, but there is little research to back that up thus far. Part of the problem is the vast array in quality within the organic subset; while an heritage tomato grown 10 miles from your house by a local farmer may be transcendent, an organic Roma tomato shipped in from Spain could leave a lot to be desired. Your best bet is to find a store or a local farmer with reliably delicious products and stick to it.

Five of the Best Salad Bar Selections

Whether your picking out ingredients for a salad at the supermarket, or faced with a dizzying array of options at your local sandwich shop, it pays to have a few nutritional star players in mind. Here are our favourites:

① SPINACH
Pick darker greens for your salad base. Spinach, on the greenest side of the spectrum, has more vitamins and nutrients than can fit on this page, including folate, which helps ward off mental decline, and beta-carotene, which helps protect your eyes and skin. It's much better than iceberg lettuce. . Its high water content makes for a low nutrient density.

② CHICKPEAS
Like all legumes, chickpeas are packed with protein and fibre, which will make you feel full. Add to that a healthy dose of antioxidants and you have the makings of a salad-topping superstar.

③ TOMATOES
Throw some the antioxidant lycopene, which has been linked to reduced risk of cancer and heart disease. Tomatoes also provide vitamins A, C, and K. They're a much better way to add sweetness than raisins, which are high in sugar.

④ AVOCADOS
These green wonders provide a ton of heart-healthy fats and a rich, creamy bite to any salad. But just because monounsaturated fats are good for your heart doesn't mean they won't still make you fat. If you choose avocados then leave out any nuts.

⑤ ALFALFA SPROUTS
These feathery salad additions have a cache of vitamins unrivalled by nearly anything else you can put in your body. Get in the habit of topping off your salad with these. Wondering what to ditch in favour of them. Sweet corn is fairly low on nutrition, so it's a common salad additive you can safely do without.

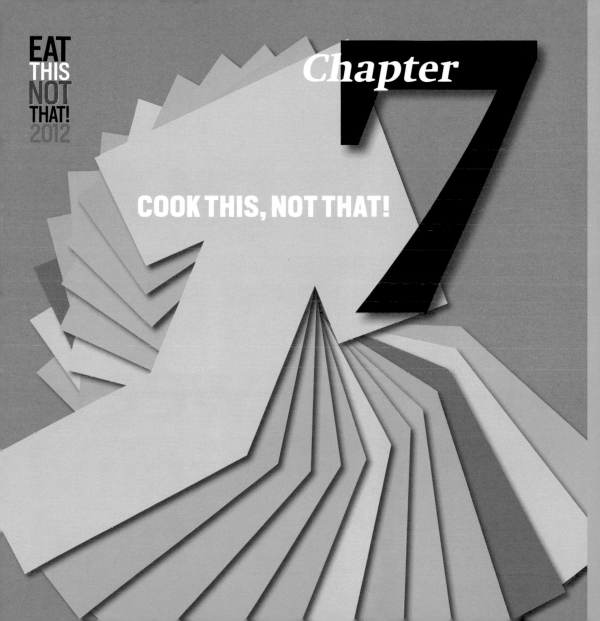

Chapter

7

COOK THIS, NOT THAT!

We know a long day. A long week. We understand that you're tired.

it's been

BUT SINCE WHEN did a ready meal taste as good as something you cooked yourself? And since when were they the most economical way to buy your food? Ready meals should be your once-in-a-while get-out-of-jail free card, not your default setting. They're expensive and often loaded with unnecessary extra salt and sugar. If you want to hand control of exactly what goes onto your plate to a multinational food corporation, day in, day out, then go ahead and pierce the film lid. If however, you'd rather save money and lose weight on a daily basis, this chapter will help you to cook up a storm, and show you exactly how much better for

you each dish is, when compared to its ready meal equivalent.

What's more, the recipes here are so simple, you'll still have plenty of time to kick back after a hard day. The average meal in this chapter takes approximately 17 minutes to prepare and costs £1.70 per serving. You don't even have to use these recipes every day to see the benefits. Fire up your cooker just three times week to make one of these dishes and, on average, you and everyone at the table will drop over half a stone this year. Not bad.

Oh, and one last piece of motivation for experimenting with these dishes: they're all completely delicious.

Breakfast Pizzas

We've seen every kind of pizza imaginable—Indian pizza, Thai chicken pizza, meatball pizza—but, surprisingly enough, no breakfast pizza. Befuddling, given just how easy and tasty it can be. Start with the ultimate breakfast bread—the fibre-dense wholemeal muffin—as your base and salsa as your sauce, then add eggs, ham, and cheese for flavour, substance, and plenty of protein. Beats a 600-calorie all day breakfast any day.

You'll Need

½ Tbsp butter

6 eggs, beaten

Salt and black pepper to taste

100 g ham, cut into thin strips

4 wholemeal muffins, split and lightly toasted

250 ml salsa

100 g grated cheddar

How To Make It

- Preheat the grill. Heat the butter in a large nonstick pan. When the butter is fully melted, season the eggs with salt and pepper, then add to the pan, along with the ham strips. Cook, using a wooden spoon or rubber spatula to keep stirring the eggs as they set.

- Remove the pan from the heat about 30 seconds before the eggs are fully done (they'll continue to cook in the pan and in the oven).

- Slather each muffin half with a good spoonful of salsa. Divide the eggs among the muffins, then top with the cheese. Place all them on a baking sheet and grill (6 inches from the heat is ideal) until the cheese is fully melted and browned around the edges.

Serves 4

$$(\overset{\text{\tiny{II}}}{\mathsf{Y}}+\mathbf{I})^2$$

MEAL MULTIPLIER

These individual pizzas have Mexican flavours at the base, but breakfast pizza can be interpreted in dozens of different ways. Here are a few other combinations (all include scrambled egg as part of the creation) that will get your day off to a rousing start:

- Pesto, mozzarella and a few slices of tomato

- Marinara sauce, provolone cheese and shredded chicken

- Guacamole, emmantal, turkey, and tomato

350 calories
19 g fat
(8 g saturated)
2.4 g salt

PER SERVING

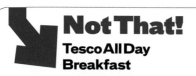

Not That!
Tesco All Day Breakfast

630 calories
33 g fat
(11.5 g saturated)
4.5 g salt

Save!
280 calories
14 g fat

248

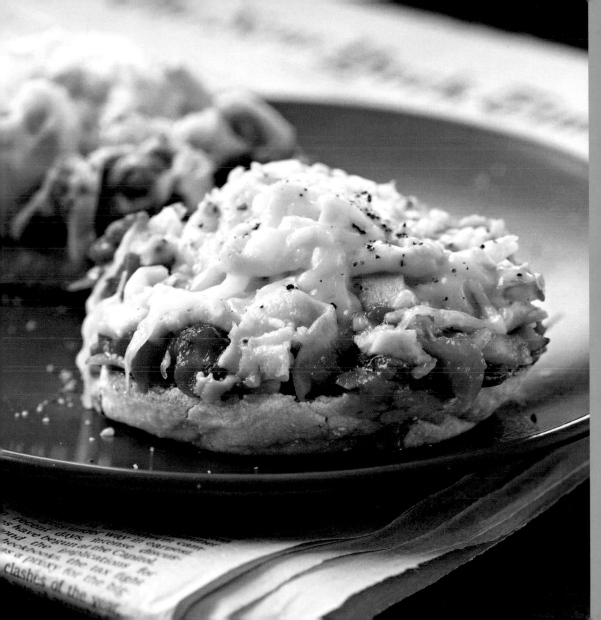

Baked Feta Cheese with Pita

Starters quite often conceal the biggest dietary dangers in the food chain. They hit us when we're at our weakest: deliriously hungry, craving greasy, fatty sustenance to the point that anything fried or covered in cheese becomes a must-have. This bubbling cheese starter has all the flavours you crave when you're hungry—salt from the olives, sweetness from the red peppers and tomatoes, fat from the cheese—but delivers them for a fraction of the calories. Serve this at your next dinner party, and when they inevitably ask for the recipe, tell them it's an old family secret.

You'll Need

240 g feta cheese
(in a single block, not crumbled)

40 g kalamata olives,
pitted and chopped

40 g chopped
sun-dried tomatoes

50 g bottled roasted red
peppers, cut into strips

Ground black pepper
to taste

1 tbsp olive oil

Juice of half a lemon

4 wholemeal pitas

How To Make It

- Preheat the oven to 190°C (gas mark 5). Place the cheese in a baking dish. Top with the olives, tomatoes, red peppers, and a sprinkle of black pepper.

- Bake until the cheese is hot and beginning to melt, about 12 to 15 minutes. Remove and drizzle with the olive oil, and squeeze the lemon over the top. While the oven is still hot, warm the pitas for a few minutes.

- Cut into quarters and serve with the cheese.

Makes 4 servings

290 calories
18 g fat
(6 g saturated)
2.4 g salt

PER SERVING

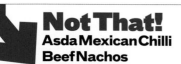

Not That!
Asda Mexican Chilli Beef Nachos

408 calories
22.5 g fat
(7.5 g saturated)
1 g salt

Save!
118 calories
4.5 g fat

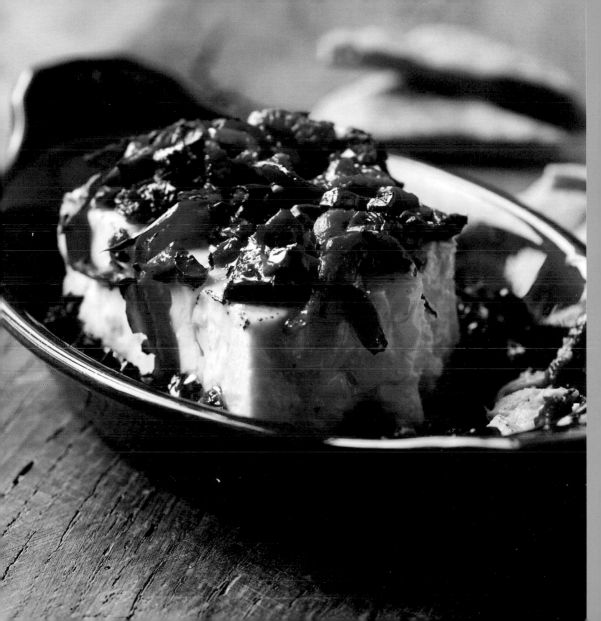

Tortilla Española

Anyone who has ever spent time in Spain will recognise this recipe as the humble national staple found on nearly every bar counter from Barcelona to Malaga, a tender omelette layered with potatoes and sweet onions. The simplicity of the ingredient list belies the depth, nuance, and soul-satisfying deliciousness a properly cooked tortilla is capable of achieving. A true Spaniard would cook the potatoes and onions in a litre of olive oil and would never use the grill to finish the cooking, but we've cut back the fat and employed the oven to make this addictive dish easier on you, and your waistline.

You'll Need

- **3 medium potatoes (about 700g), diced**
- **2 tbsp olive oil**
- **1 large onion, diced**
- **1 tsp salt**
- **8 eggs, beaten**

How To Make It

- Fill a large cast-iron skillet or 12 inch frying pan with water. Add the potatoes and bring to a boil. Cook for about 10 minutes, until the potatoes have softened but aren't completely tender. Drain.

- Preheat the grill. Return the potatoes to the same pan, along with the olive oil and onion, and cook over medium-low heat, stirring occasionally, for about 5 minutes, until the onions begin to brown and the potatoes are cooked through. Season with the salt.

- Add the eggs to the pan, cover, and cook for about 10 minutes, until most of the egg is set. Uncover and finish by placing the pan under the grill for 3 to 4 minutes to brown the top of the tortilla. Let the tortilla rest for a few minutes. When ready to eat, slip from the pan and cut into wedges.

Makes 6 servings

290 calories
10 g fat
(2.5 g saturated)
1.2 g salt

PER SERVING

Not That!
**Sainsbury's Taste
The Difference
Quiche Lorraine**

402 calories
28.3 g fat
(14.7 g saturated)
1.9 g salt

Save!

*112 calories
18.3 g fat*

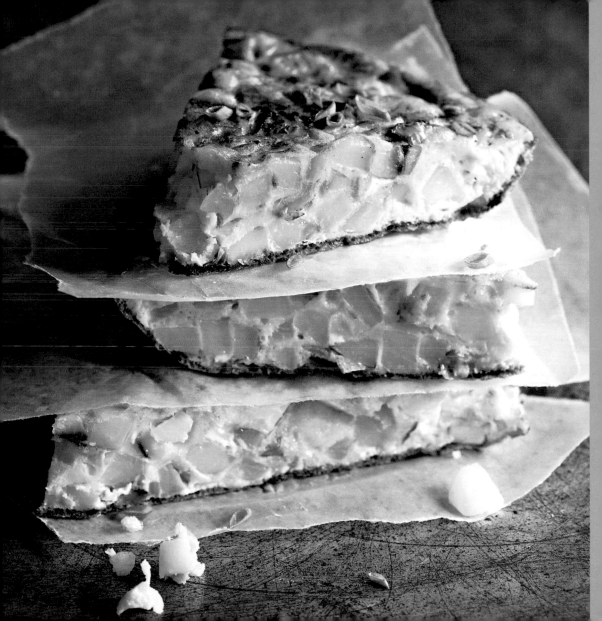

Asian Beef Salad with Sriracha-Honey Dressing

Pre-prepared salads suffer from a double dose of shamefulness: They are not only boring and sloppily executed, they often come with more calories and fat than your average bacon cheeseburger. Here, we harbour the big flavours of the East—sweet, spicy, tart, cool— but leave all the excessive calories out of the equation. A generous portion of lean flank steak and creamy cubes of avocado make sure this salad truly satisfies.

You'll Need

450 g flank steak (ask your butcher, this great-value cut is under used)

Salt and ground black pepper to taste

1 tsp sriracha or other hot sauce

2 tsp honey

½ tbsp reduced-salt soy sauce

Juice of 1 lime

60 ml canola oil

1 bag watercress

1 small punnet of cherry tomatoes, sliced in half

1 small red onion, thinly sliced

½ cucumber, thinly sliced

1 avocado, peeled, pitted, and chopped

Handful of fresh coriander leaves

How To Make It

- Preheat a grill, grill pan, or cast-iron skillet over medium-high heat. Season the flank steak all over with salt and pepper and cook until medium rare, about 3 to 4 minutes per side. Allow the steak to rest for at least 5 minutes before slicing thinly across the natural grain of the meat.

- While the meat rests, combine the sriracha, honey, soy sauce, and lime juice with a pinch of pepper in a mixing bowl. Slowly drizzle in the oil, whisking to combine.

- In a large salad bowl, combine the watercress, tomatoes, onion, cucumber, avocado, coriander, and sliced steak and slowly drizzle in the dressing, tossing the ingredients gently with each addition, until everything is lightly coated.

Makes 4 servings

430 calories
31 g fat
(6 g saturated)
1.14 g salt

PER SERVING

600 calories
40 g fat
(4 g saturated)
1.4 g salt

Save!
170 calories
9 g fat

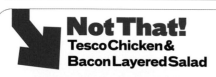

Not That!
Tesco Chicken & Bacon Layered Salad

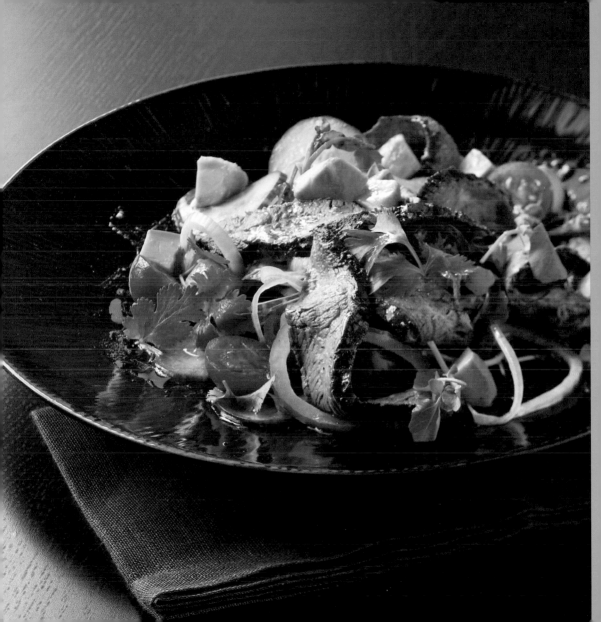

Minestrone with Pesto

Nearly 9 out of 10 Britons don't consume enough fruit and vegetables on a daily basis. This soup will go a long way to making sure you're not one of them. Vary the specific vegetables depending on what's in your fridge and what looks good in the market, but be sure to finish with a spoonful of pesto sauce, which helps tie the whole bowl together.

$$(\text{Y+1})^2$$

MEAL MULTIPLIER

The best part about minestrone is that the same basic technique can be applied to nearly any combination of vegetables. Change up this recipe depending on the season, keeping the onion, garlic, potatoes, pesto, tomatoes, and stock intact but adding one of these timely teams:

- Autumn: Cubed butternut squash and halved Brussels sprouts

- Winter: Chopped Swiss chard, shredded cabbage, and chopped celery

- Spring: Start with cauliflower, then add asparagus and green peas or broad beans in the final minutes before serving

You'll Need

1 tbsp olive oil

1 medium onion, chopped

2 cloves garlic, crushed

220 g red potatoes, cubed

2 medium carrots, peeled and chopped

1 medium courgette, chopped

220 g green beans, ends trimmed, halved

Salt and black pepper to taste

1 tin chopped tomatoes

2 litres low-salt chicken stock (or a mixture of stock and water)

½ tsp dried thyme

½ tin white beans (eg cannellini), drained

Pesto

Parmesan for grating

How To Make It

- Heat the olive oil in a large pot over medium heat. Add the onion and garlic and cook until the onion is translucent, about 3 minutes. Stir in the potatoes, carrots, courgette, and green beans. Season with a bit of salt and cook, stirring, for 3 to 4 minutes to release the vegetables' aromas. Add the tomatoes, stock, and thyme and turn the heat down to low. Season with salt (if still needed) and pepper to taste. Simmer for at least 15 minutes, and up to 45.

- Before serving, stir in the white beans and heat through. Serve with a dollop of pesto and bit of grated Parmesan.

Makes 4 servings

200 calories
5 g fat
(1.5 g saturated)
1.2 g salt

PER SERVING

347 calories
13.1 g fat
(5.1 g saturated)
2.4 g salt

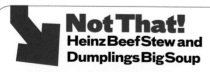

Not That!
Heinz Beef Stew and Dumplings Big Soup

Save!
*147 calories
8.1 g fat*

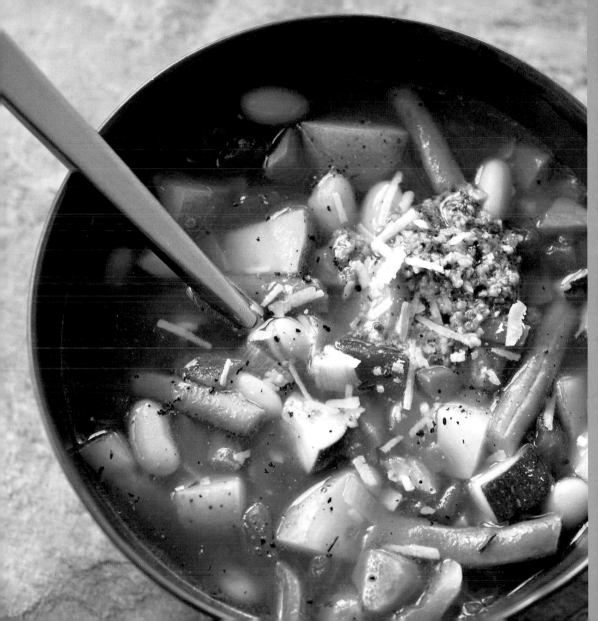

Cook This!
Turkey & Brie with Apple

It's a pretty simple concept: The more stuffed full a sandwich, the more calories it will contain. This holds true time and time again in the takeaway world, where concepts rife with potential, go down in a burst of flames once bedecked with bells and whistles. It doesn't have to be that way. We've used add-ons to the greater good of this handheld wonder: Slices of apple add coolness and crunch; a quick honey-mustard mix provides sweetness and spice; and a few slices of brie bring that intense creaminess we all crave. All told, the condiment treatment here tacks onto the sandwich about 100 calories—not bad for a trio that also bolsters fibre, antioxidants, and, above all, flavour.

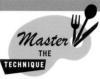

Master THE TECHNIQUE

Sweet and Savoury Sandwiches

Nothing wrong with standard turkey, ham, or roast beef, but we like to push the culinary boundaries in the sandwich genre. A favourite technique is to pair savoury meats with sweet fruits to create a yin-yang balance that will keep your taste buds at full attention. Here's a few of our favourites:

- Prosciutto or other good ham with sliced figs and crumbled goat cheese

- Grilled chicken, grilled pineapple, and melted cheese

- Peanut butter, banana, and crispy bacon (Elvis has never steered us wrong!)

You'll Need

- 2 tbsp plain mustard
- 2 tbsp honey
- 4 seeded wholemeal rolls, split and lightly toasted
- 1 apple, thinly sliced
- 4 handfuls baby spinach
- 4 thin slices red onion
- 450 g sliced smoked turkey
- 60 g brie cheese, thinly sliced

How To Make It

- Combine the mustard and honey in a small bowl and spread on the bottom half of each roll. Divide the apple among the rolls, then top with the divided spinach, red onion, turkey, and cheese.

Makes 4 sandwiches

410 calories
10 g fat
(4 g saturated)
2.2 g salt

PER SERVING

567 calories
33.3 g fat
(11.9 g saturated)
1.9 g salt

Save!
157 calories
23.3 g fat

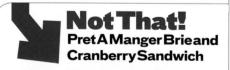

Not That!
Pret A Manger Brie and Cranberry Sandwich

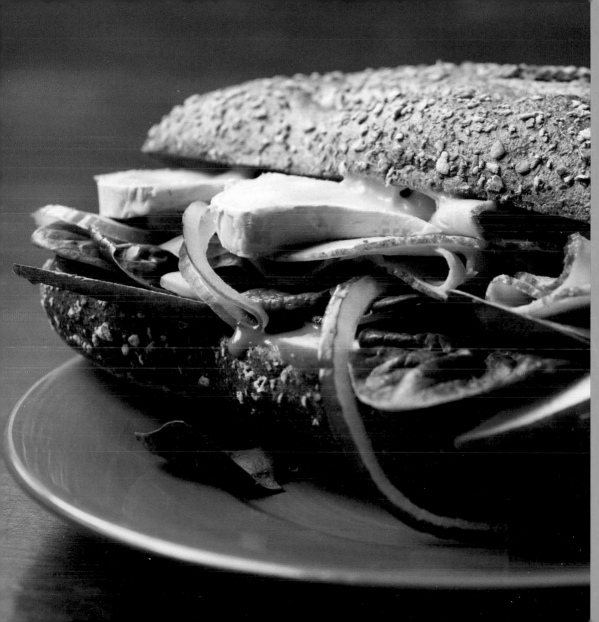

Roasted Halibut
Wrapped in Prosciutto

The traditional British way to cook fish (wrapped in batter and deep fried) is, you won't be surprised to learn, not exactly what we'd call healthy. Even if you opt for an innocent looking fish cake you can be caught out by added potato and sauces. We skip the crusting and frying and instead opt for a simpler, healthier, and (we think) more delicious alternative: wrapping. It looks fancy and tastes like a sophisticated fine-dining dish, but the truth is that this is the simplest recipe in this chapter.

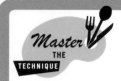

Master THE TECHNIQUE

Wrapping Fish and Meat

Rather than smothering meat or fish with viscous, calorie-dense sauces or, worse yet, deep-frying it, encasing it in a thin sheet of prosciutto or Spanish-style *jamón* is an excellent way to keep the flesh moist and tender without adding more than 50 calories to the final dish. Place a chicken breast, pork loin, or meaty fish fillet in the centre of a strip of prosciutto, season with salt and pepper, and wrap tightly. Roast on a baking tray in the oven until cooked all the way through.

You'll Need

- **4 pieces (170g each) halibut, cod, sea bass, or other flaky white fish**
- **Salt and ground black pepper to taste**
- **4 thin slices prosciutto**
- **1 lemon, quartered**
- **2 tbsp prepared pesto**

How To Make It

- Preheat the oven to 190°C/gas mark 5. Season the fish all over with salt and pepper. Lay the slices of prosciutto on a cutting board and wrap each piece of fish tightly with one of the slices. Place the fish on a baking tray and position it on the middle rack of the oven. Roast until the prosciutto begins to crisp up and the fish flakes with gentle pressure from your finger, about 10 to 12 minutes. Serve each with a wedge of lemon and the pesto drizzled over the top.

Makes 4 servings

230 calories
8 g fat
(2 g saturated)
1.4 g salt

PER SERVING

316 calories
15.6 g fat
(5.8 g saturated)
1.2 g salt

Save!
86 calories
7.6 g fat

Not That!
Asda Extra Special Oven-Baked Smoked Haddock fishcakes

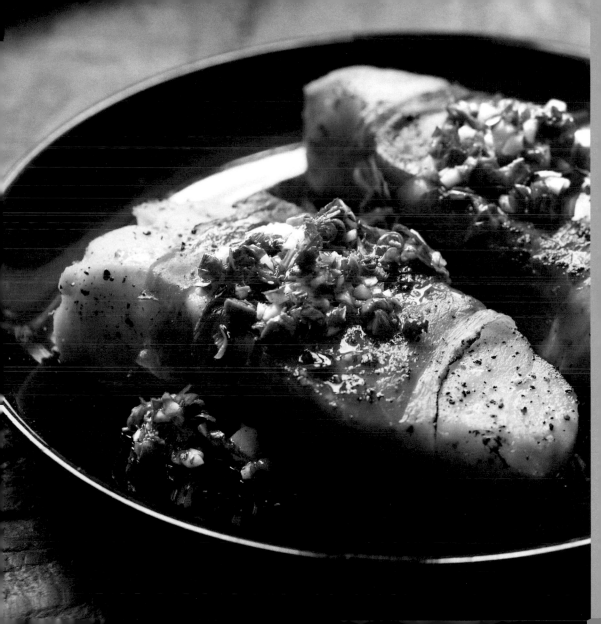

Chickpeas
with Chorizo and Spinach

The Spanish have one of the longest life spans on the planet, and when you look at their eating habits, it's not hard to see why. Meat plays a secondary role to fish and vegetables, often being used as a supporting actor rather than the star of the dish. That's the philosophy behind this classic stew, which uses a few chunks of chorizo to infuse an entire pot of fibre-rich chickpeas and wilted spinach with smoky, meaty flavour.

You'll Need

- ½ tbsp olive oil
- 2 links chorizo, chopped
- 1 large onion, chopped
- 2 cloves garlic, minced
- ¼ tsp dried red pepper flakes
- 1 tsp paprika
- 2 bay leaves
- 2 tbsp tomato paste
- 500 g potatoes, cut into ½-inch chunks
- 350 ml low-salt chicken stock
- Salt and ground black pepper to taste
- 2 tins (400 g) chickpeas, drained and rinsed
- 8 handfuls baby spinach

How To Make It

- Heat the oil in a large pot or saucepan over medium heat. Add the chorizo and sauté until the meat is lightly browned. Move to a plate and reserve.

- Add the onion, garlic, red pepper flakes, paprika, and bay leaves to the pan and cook until the onion begins to brown, about 5 minutes. Stir in the tomato paste and cook for another few minutes, until it evenly coats the onions and garlic. Add the potatoes and stock, and simmer the vegetables until the potatoes are just tender, about 10 minutes. Add the chickpeas and cook for another 5 minutes. Season with salt and black pepper to taste.

- Just before you're ready to serve, stir in the reserved chorizo and the spinach and cook until the spinach wilts.

Makes 6 servings

SECRET WEAPON
Chorizo

Look out for some genuine Spanish chorizo, which is cured, but derives most of its flavour (and colour) from smoked paprika, for this dish. While other types of sausage will work Spanish chorizo is really what you're looking for here. A few hunks sautéed with onions and garlic form a brilliant base for a pot of black beans, lentils, chilli, or even scrambled eggs. Just go easy with it. You only need a little to flavour a whole dish and it has a high fat content, so it's worth treating with respect.

360 calories
11 g fat
(3.5 g saturated)
2 g salt

PER SERVING

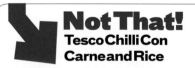

Not That!
Tesco Chilli Con Carne and Rice

540 calories
10.4 g fat
(3.6 g saturated)
2 g salt

Save!
180 calories
0.6g fat

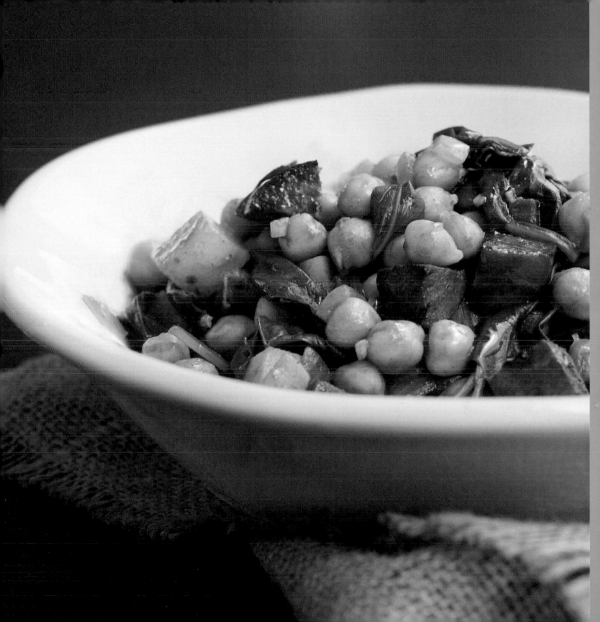

Sausage Penne Courgette and Goat's Cheese

Pasta has had a bad rap of late, what with Dr Atkins and the low-carb crowd. The truth is, it's a healthy low-fat way to boost energy levels. Pasta only becomes unhealthy when served with the creamy sauces and fatty meats that are often found in supermarket ready meals. Our answer? A low-calorie, big-flavour dish that packs an energy punch and that you can pack for lunch.

You'll Need

340 g penne pasta

1 tbsp olive oil

220 g uncooked chicken sausages, skin removed

1 medium onion, chopped

2 cloves garlic, thinly sliced

1 medium courgette, sliced into half-moons

Salt and ground black pepper to taste

40 g sun-dried tomatoes, reconstituted in hot water if not oil-packed

120 ml chicken stock

45 g goat cheese

How To Make It

● Bring a large pot of generously salted water to a boil and cook the pasta until just *al dente*, meaning 'hard bite'. As always, rely on your taste buds—not the package instructions—to determine this.

● While the water heats and the pasta cooks, heat the oil in a large frying pan over medium-high heat. Add the sausage and fry until cooked all the way through, about 5 minutes. Remove and reserve. Add the onion and garlic and cook for a few minutes, until the onion is translucent, then add the courgette and cook until lightly caramelised, about 5 more minutes. Season with salt and pepper. Add the sun-dried tomatoes, the stock, and the reserved sausage and keep warm until the pasta is ready.

● Drain the pasta and add it directly to the pan with the sausage and vegetables. Cook together for 30 seconds, cut the heat, and sprinkle on the cheese just before serving.

Makes 4 servings

480 calories
11 g fat
(4 g saturated)
1.5 g salt

PER SERVING

Not That!
Tesco Finest Chicken and Beech Smoked Bacon Pasta Bake

681 calories
31.2 g fat
(16.8 g saturated)
2.6 g salt

Save!
201 calories
20.2g fat

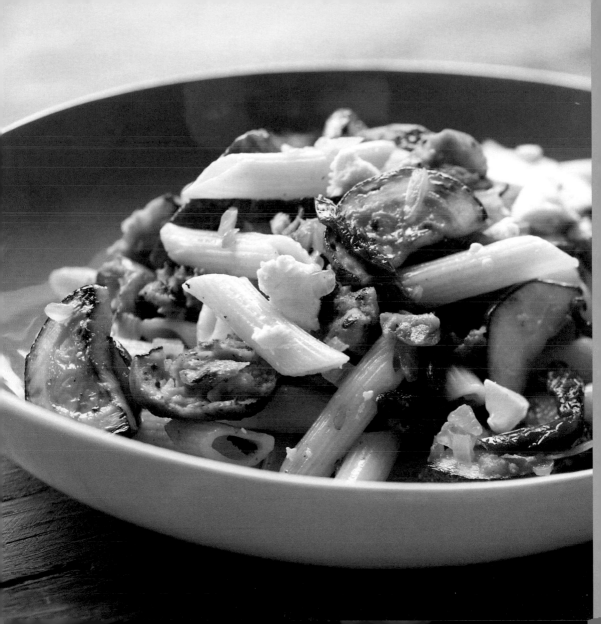

Greek Chicken with Lemon-Yogurt Sauce

Grilled chicken is one of those great barbecue dishes that needs very little help. Fire up the outdoor grill (charcoal, preferably, but gas will do), add some salt and pepper, and cook until the skin is lightly charred and smoky and the meat is moist and tender. It's a back garden miracle, re-created year after year. We don't want to tweak the formula too much, but with a simple marinade and a 1-minute sauce, you can turn a dish that's consistently good into something truly magical.

You'll Need

240 ml low-fat Greek yogurt

6 cloves garlic, minced and divided

Juice of two lemons, divided

3 tbsp olive oil, divided

1 kg bone-in, skin-on chicken thighs and drumsticks

1 tsp dried oregano

Big pinch salt and grind of black pepper to taste

How To Make It

- Combine the yogurt, one-third of the garlic, the juice of half a lemon, and 1 tablespoon of the olive oil. Mix thoroughly and reserve in the refrigerator.

- Combine the chicken with the oregano, salt, pepper, and the remaining garlic, lemon juice, and olive oil. Cover and marinate in the refrigerator for at least 30 minutes and up to 4 hours.

- Preheat a grill or grill pan. Remove the chicken from the marinade and grill over a medium flame until the skin is nicely caramelised and the meat is cooked all the way through, about 15 to 20 minutes. Serve with the yogurt on the side or drizzled over the top.

Makes 4 servings

SECRET WEAPON

Chicken Skin

Popular belief has it that chicken skin is flat-out bad for you. Indeed, many prominent nutritionists and organisations (including the American Heart Association) continue to regurgitate the antiquated mantra that all animal fat is bad for you, despite reams of evidence suggesting otherwise. Despite its reputation, chicken skin contains a heavy dose of mono-unsaturated oleic acid, the very same heart-healthy kind you find in olive oil. Still, calories come with fat, and if cutting calories is your first priority, grill the chicken with the skin on (it will keep the meat moist and tender), then remove it before eating.

395 calories
30 g fat
(7 g saturated)
0.5 g salt

PER SERVING

472 calories
32 g fat
(10.7 g saturated)
0.7 g salt

Not That!
Waitrose Chicken Crown with Lemon Tarragon and Shallots

Save!
77 calories
3.7 g sat fat

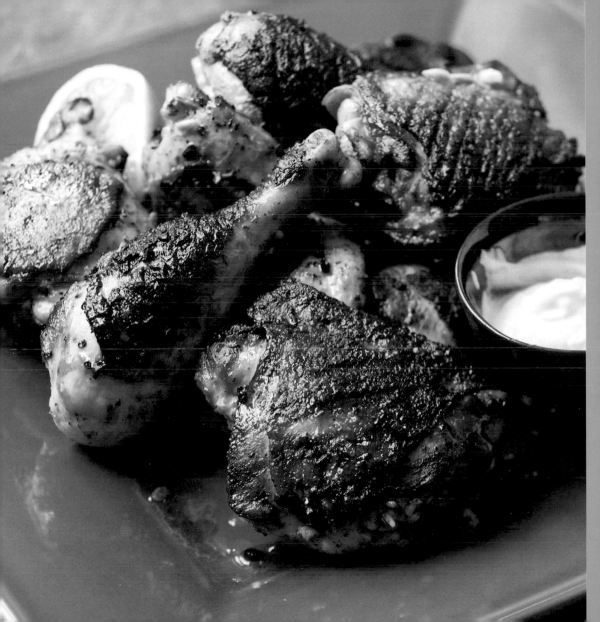

Lasagne Rolls

The idea of building a multi-tiered, multi-component lasagne can be dizzying for most cooks. For them, we offer this simplified form, the lasagne roll: a tight pasta bundle containing all the same flavours, but without the daunting architecture. It's basic shape helps you avoid creating one of those cheesy, soupy catastrophes so common in restaurants, the ones where it's impossible to discern where the pasta stops and the sauce begins. The structure is sound, the flavours are clear and pronounced, and the calories are greatly reduced. What more could you want?

You'll Need

10-12 long, thin lasagne

170 g chicken sausage, skin removed

1 bag frozen spinach, thawed

¼ tsp red pepper flakes

Pinch of nutmeg

Salt and black pepper to taste

45 g low-fat ricotta cheese

500 g jar marinara pasta sauce

30 g grated low-fat mozzarella

How To Make It

• Bring a large pot of salted water to a boil. Add the lasagne and cook until al dente (usually about 30 seconds to a minute less than the package instructions). Drain and toss with just enough oil to coat (to keep them from sticking).

• While the pasta cooks, brown the sausage in a large sauté pan over medium heat until cooked through. Add the spinach, pepper flakes, and nutmeg and cook until the spinach is warmed through. Season with salt and pepper. Remove from heat and let cool slightly. Combine with the ricotta in a large mixing bowl.

• Preheat the oven to 200°C/gas mark 6. Spread a thin layer of the marinara on the bottom of a baking dish. Lay out the pasta on a cutting board and cut each in half crossways. Working one strip at a time, place a large spoonful of the spinach-ricotta mixture at the end of the noodle, then roll into a tight package (but not too tight or the filling will squeeze out). Continue until you've run out of the ricotta-spinach mixture, about 20 lasagne rolls. Place the rolls in the pan as you complete each one.

• Top the lasagne rolls with the remaining marinara, then with the mozzarella. Cover with foil and bake for 15 minutes. Remove the foil and bake for another 10 minutes, until the cheese and sauce are bubbling.

Makes 6 servings

380 calories
11 g fat
(3.5 g saturated)
2 g salt

PER SERVING

Not That!
Waitrose Beef Lasagne

473 calories
22.4 g fat
(8.9 g saturated)
2.2 g salt

Save!
93 calories
11.4 g fat

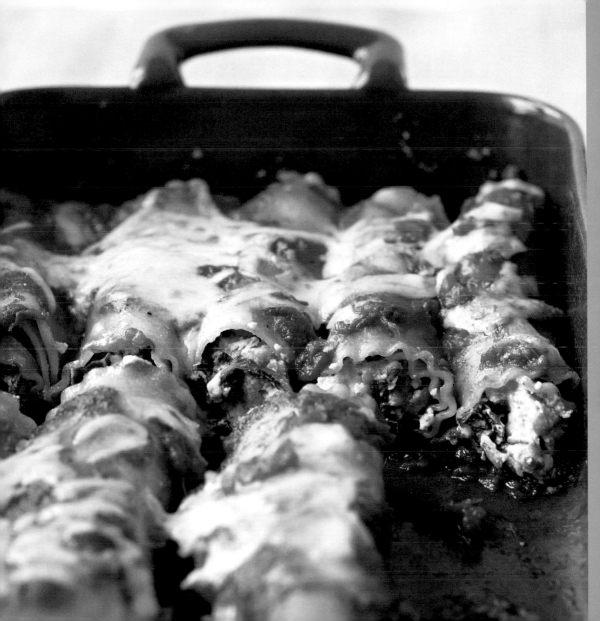

Hoisin Beef Kebab

In the Shinjuku district of Tokyo, behind the central train station (the busiest in the world), you'll find a long, narrow alleyway—appropriately dubbed Yakitori Alley—that is lined with dozens of tiny bars and stands billowing savoury smoke into the air. Humble grill masters expertly char skewered food of all shapes and sizes: plump meatballs, tiny cherry tomatoes, even pure chicken skin that crisps up like potato chips. Though we never had this exact kebab there, the flavours are true to the spirit of Yakitori Alley; we hope the grill masters would approve.

You'll Need

- 2 tbsp hoisin sauce
- 1 tbsp low-salt soy sauce
- 2 tsp dark or toasted sesame oil
- 1 tsp chili sauce or paste, such as sriracha
- 500 g sirloin, cut into 2 cm pieces
- 8 spring onion whites
- 20 small mushrooms
- 20 cherry tomatoes
- 8 wooden skewers, soaked in water for 20 minutes

How To Make It

- Preheat a grill. Combine the hoisin, soy sauce, sesame oil, and chilli sauce in a bowl and mix. Transfer half to a separate bowl and reserve.

- Thread the beef, spring onions, mushrooms, and cherry tomatoes onto the skewers, alternating meat and vegetables. Use a brush to paint the skewers with the remaining hoisin glaze. When the grill (or griddle pan) is hot, add the skewers and cook for 3 to 4 minutes per side, basting with sauce as you go. The skewers are done when the meat and vegetables are lightly charred and the beef is firm but still yielding to the touch.

- Brush the kebabs with the reserved glaze before serving.

Serves 4

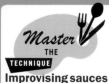

Master THE TECHNIQUE

Improvising sauces

Making a killer sauce for the grill on the fly is easier than most think. Start with a base with a well-rounded flavour: ketchup, Dijon and hoisin all work. Then mix in other liquids or condiments that add strong single flavour notes: honey for sweetness, vinegar for acid, soy sauce for salt, sriracha for heat. Finally, turn to the spice cabinet to bring it all together. Chilli powder, garlic and onion salt, cumin, brown sugar, mustard powder, and cayenne are all common elements when you're grilling meat and could be the finishing touch for your next masterpiece.

290 calories
10 g fat
(3 g saturated)
2.17 g salt

PER SERVING

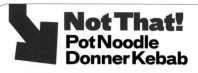

Not That!
Pot Noodle Donner Kebab

413 calories
16.3 g fat
(6.8 g saturated)
1.85 g salt

Save!
123 calories
6.3 g fat

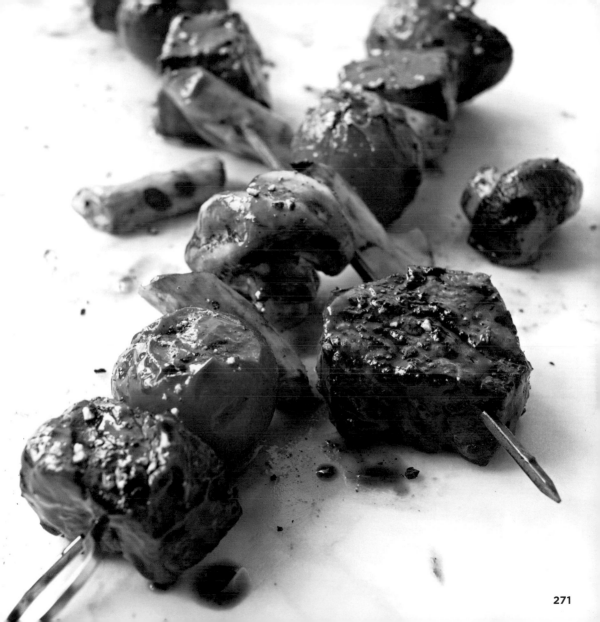

Chicken under a Brick

Drop the bottled barbecue sauce! The Italians have a magical way to barbecue chicken that involves no special sauces or condiments; in fact, all you really need is a brick or two and some aluminum foil. Whoever first placed brick to backbone was smart enough to recognise that the extra weight helped press the bird evenly—and forcefully—against the grill, which translates into a juicier bird with a crisper skin—a win-win in our book.

You'll Need

60 ml olive oil

Grated zest and juice of 1 lemon

1 tsp red pepper flakes

1 tsp salt

½ tsp black pepper

1 whole chicken, back removed, split in half

2 lemons, halved

2 bricks, covered in aluminum foil

How To Make It

- Combine the olive oil, lemon zest and juice, pepper flakes, salt, and pepper in a large bowl, baking dish, or resealable plastic bag. Add the chicken and turn to coat. Cover the bowl or seal the bag and marinate in the refrigerator for at least 30 minutes and up to 4 hours.

- Fire up your barbecue (you want a nice medium-low heat). Remove the chicken from the marinade and place on the grate, skin side up. Cover in foil and cook for 10 minutes, until the chicken is lightly charred. Flip the chicken over, then place a brick on top of each half so that it presses the chicken firmly and evenly against the grate. Cook for another 15 to 20 minutes, until the skin is thoroughly browned and crisp and the meat pulls away easily from the bone. (If the barbecue flares up, move the chicken to a cooler part of the grill.) While the chicken cooks, toss on the lemon halves, cut side down, and grill until charred and juicy.

- Separate each breast from the chicken leg by making a cut right at the thigh bone. Serve each of the four pieces of chicken with a grilled lemon half.

Serves 4

Master **THE** `TECHNIQUE`

Brick cooking

It may be the crudest, most rudimentary of tools, but a sturdy, foil-wrapped brick comes in handy in the kitchen. Try placing it on top of a pork chop or a flank steak in a cast-iron pan—the extra pressure will yield a beautifully caramelized crust. Better yet, it's perfect for making a panini: Simply place the sandwich in a hot cast-iron skillet, top with a brick, cook for 2 or 3 minutes, then flip and repeat.

280 calories
8 g fat
(2 g saturated)
1.95 g salt

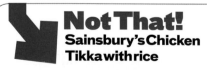

Not That!
Sainsbury's Chicken Tikka with rice

819 calories
33 g fat
(10.5 g saturated)
2.77 g salt

Save!
539 calories
25 g fat

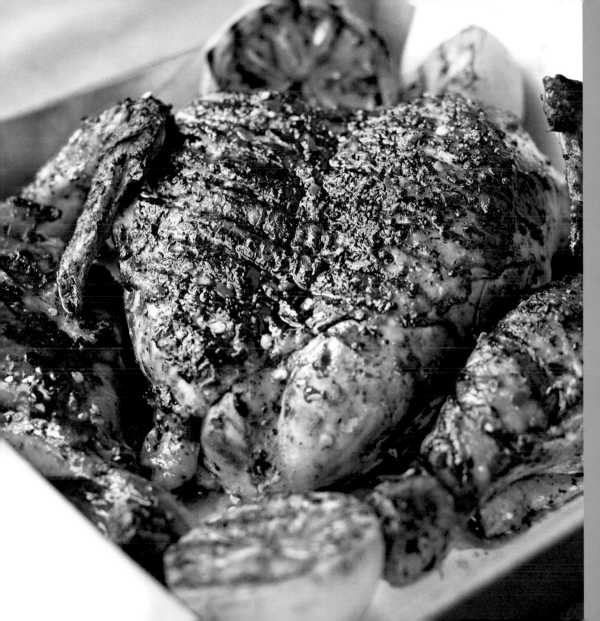

Bloody Mary Steak

As delicious as a Bloody Mary is as a drink, it makes an even better marinade. That's because the mix of sweet and salty from the tomato juice, the heat from the horseradish and Tabasco, and the acid from the lemon work together to both tenderise and energise an otherwise normal piece of beef. This marinade could do magic on chicken and pork as well, but the bold flavours of a Bloody seem to pair best with a hunk of grilled beef. Serve with grilled asparagus and roasted potatoes for a near-perfect meal.

You'll Need

500 ml tomato juice

2 tbsp prepared horseradish

4 cloves garlic, minced

Juice of 1 lemon

½ tbsp Worcestershire sauce

10–15 shakes Tabasco sauce

Black pepper to taste

500 g lean steak

How To Make It

- Combine the tomato juice, horseradish, garlic, lemon juice, Worcestershire, Tabasco, and pepper in a baking dish and use a whisk to thoroughly mix (on this occasion you can leave out the vodka).

- If your steak is quite thick (more than a couple of centimetres) bash it out a little with a kitchen mallet or with your fist. Then add the steak to the marinade and turn it over several times to coat it completely in the mixture. Cover with cling film. Put the whole dish in the refrigerator to marinate for at least 2 hours or up to 12.

- Preheat a grill. Pour off the marinade and discard. Use a paper kitchen towel to pat most of the marinade from the steak.

- When the grill is very hot, add the steak and cook for a couple of minutes per side for medium rare.

- Let the meat rest for at least 5 minutes before cutting into thin slices against the grain of the meat to serve.

Serves 4

270 calories
11 g fat
(4.5 g saturated)
1.13 g salt

PER SERVING

471 calories
32 g fat
(13 g saturated)
1.75 g salt

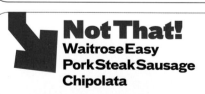

Not That!
Waitrose Easy Pork Steak Sausage Chipolata

Save!
201 calories
21 g fat

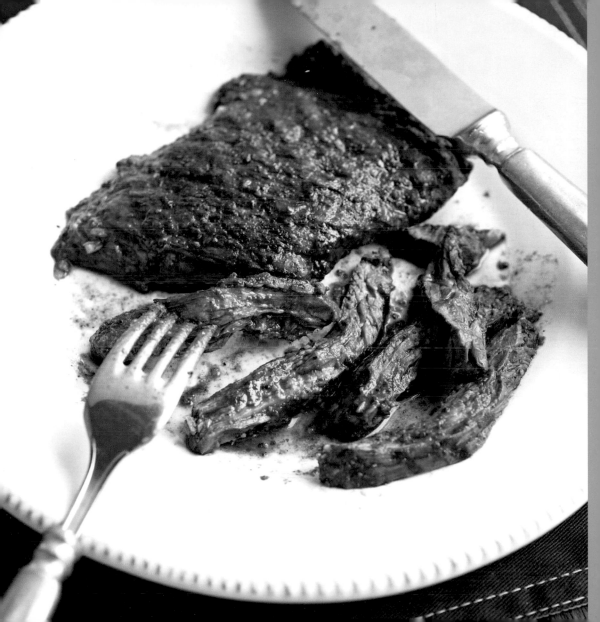

Cook This!
Crispy Duck Breast with Balsamic Cherries

Like lamb, buffalo, and rabbit, duck gets no love from the home cook. Problem is, duck is viewed as complicated food; a fancy ingredient that requires a deft touch to prepare. Not so. All it takes is a hot pan and a bit of salt and pepper to cook up a moist, juicy duck breast that will rival any supermarket steak. Seven ingredients and 15 minutes is all you need.

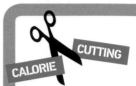

CALORIE CUTTING

You'll Need

4 small duck breasts or 2 large breasts (about 500 g total)

Salt and black pepper to taste

2 shallots, minced

16 cherries, pitted and roughly chopped

60 ml low-sodium chicken stock

60 ml balsamic vinegar

How To Make It

- Heat a griddle pan over medium heat. Use a sharp knife to score the skin on each duck breast, cutting ½ inch diamonds across the entire surface. Season all over with salt and black pepper. Add the duck breasts to the pan, skin side down, and cook for 5 to 6 minutes, until plenty of fat has rendered and the skin is a deep golden brown. Flip and cook for another 3 to 4 minutes, until the duck is firm but yielding. Transfer to a cutting board and let rest for 5 minutes.

- While the duck rests, discard all but a thin film of the duck fat. (If you really want to indulge, roast some potatoes in the fat tomorrow.) Add the shallots to the pan and cook for 1 minute before adding the cherries. Cook for 2 minutes, then pour in the stock and vinegar. Simmer for about 3 minutes, until the liquid has reduced by half. Season with black pepper.

- Thinly slice the duck and divide among four plates. Serve with the cherry-balsamic sauce spooned over the top.

Serves 4

Take comfort in the fact that most of the duck's fat is healthy fat. But healthy or not, every kind of fat, regardless of source, packs 9 calories per gram, more than twice what you'd take in from a gram of carbs or protein. If you're looking to take this dish as low as it goes, simply follow the recipe, but after the duck has rested on the cutting board, use a knife to cut away the top layer of crispy fat. Why not remove it before cooking? Because it will help insulate and baste the breast while it cooks, leaving you with juicier meat, even after the fat is gone.

270 calories
10 g fat
(3 g saturated)
0.72 g salt

PER SERVING

440 calories
16.8 g fat
(4.4 g saturated)
2.2 g salt

Not That!
Asda Shredded Duck Meal

Save!
170 calories
6.8 g fat

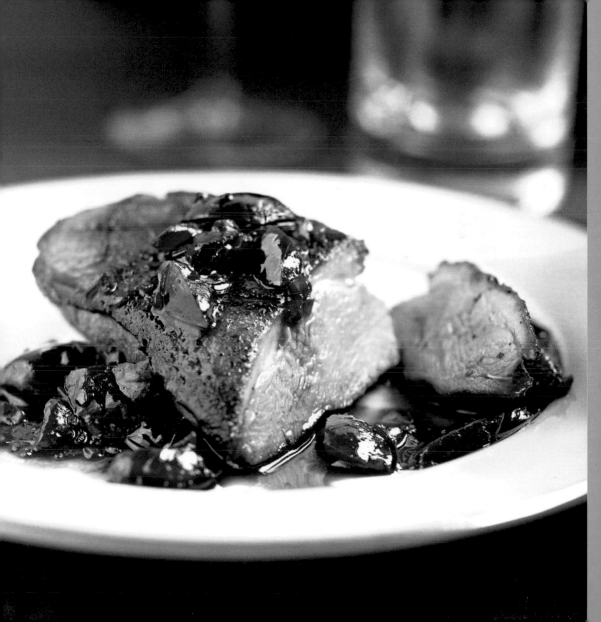

Grilled Calamari Salad

Squid is one of the most abundant forms of seafood, yet few Brits have ever enjoyed it in any other way than breaded and deep-fried. With that type of treatment, it could be an onion ring and you wouldn't know the difference. This salad has all the trappings of the much-adored appetiser—crunch from the peanuts, tomatoes, a bit of spice—but so much more. We don't want to promise that you'll never go back to the fried stuff after this, but it's a distinct possibility.

You'll Need

450 g squid, cleaned

½ tbsp peanut or canola oil

Salt and black pepper to taste

Juice of 1 lime

1 tbsp fish sauce

1 tbsp sugar

½ tbsp chili garlic sauce (preferably sambal oleek)

4 handfuls of watercress

1 small cucumber, peeled, seeded, and cut into matchsticks

1 medium tomato, chopped

½ red onion, very thinly sliced

30 g cup roasted peanuts

How To Make It

- Preheat a grill. Toss the squid bodies with the oil and generously season with salt and lots of black pepper. When the grill is very hot, add the squid and grill for about 5 minutes, until lightly charred all over.

- Combine the lime juice, fish sauce, sugar, and chilli sauce in a mixing bowl and whisk to blend. Slice the grilled squid into ½ inch rings. In a salad bowl, toss the squid, watercress, cucumber, tomato, onion, and peanuts with the dressing. Divide the salad among 4 plates.

Serves 4

Master
THE
TECHNIQUE

Cooking calamari

Grilling squid ranks right up there next to tying your shoes and making your bed in difficulty, yet most people are terrified of the prospect. Purchase whole squid bodies (available fully cleaned, fresh or frozen, at any decent fish market or quality grocery store) and either grill them whole over high heat for no more than 5 minutes, or cut them into rings and sauté in olive oil for the same amount of time.

220 calories
8 g fat
(1.5 g saturated)
1.4 g salt

PER SERVING

384 calories
3.3 g fat
(2 g saturated)
1.5 g salt

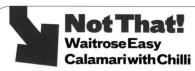

Not That!
Waitrose Easy
Calamari with Chilli

Save!
164 calories
0.5 g sat fat

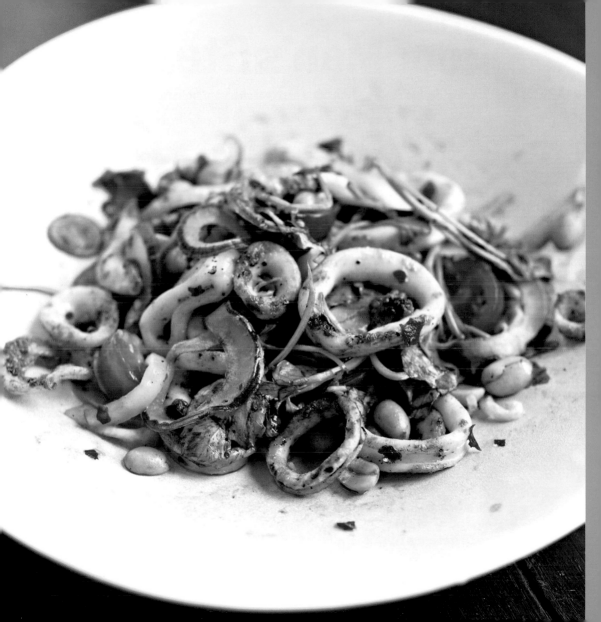

Poor Man's Steak with Garlic Gravy

This country has fallen on lean times in recent years, but unfortunately the figurative belt-tightening doesn't seem to be accompanied by a literal one. That's because the most potent sources of calories and seasoning (oil, butter, sugar, salt) are still cheap and more common in cooking than ever. Here, we mimic its taste and tenderness with inexpensive lean, minced beef and cover it with a soy-spiked sauce good enough to make your doormat taste delicious. Serve this hot, decadent mess over a velvety bed of mashed potatoes, or for a healthier, easier sidekick, try spinach sautéed in olive oil and chopped garlic.

You'll Need

450 g minced lean beef shaped into 4 equal patties

1 tbsp canola oil

Salt and ground black pepper to taste

2 cloves garlic, minced

1 onion, sliced

100 g white mushrooms, stems removed, sliced

½ tbsp flour

120 ml beef or chicken stock

1 tbsp ketchup

1 tbsp reduced salt soy sauce

1 tsp Worcestershire sauce

How to Make It

- Preheat the oven to 135°C/gas mark 1.
- Heat a large cast-iron skillet or frying pan over medium-high heat. Season the patties all over with salt and pepper. Add the oil to the pan and cook until a nicely browned crust forms on the patties, about 3 to 4 minutes, then flip and continue cooking for another 3 to 4 minutes for medium-rare. Move the patties to a baking tray and place in the oven to keep warm.
- Add the remaining oil and the garlic, onions, and mushrooms to the same pan, and cook until the vegetables begin to brown nicely, about 5 to 7 minutes. Sprinkle the flour over the vegetables, stir so that it coats them evenly, then add the stock, using a whisk to keep lumps from forming. Stir in the ketchup, soy sauce, and Worcestershire sauce and continue cooking until the gravy thickens, another 2 to 3 minutes. Serve the patties on a bed of mashed potatoes or sautéed spinach (or both) with the gravy drizzled over the top.

Makes 4 servings

220 calories
9 g fat
(3 g saturated)
1.2 g salt

PER SERVING

569 calories
25.4 g fat
(11.2 g saturated)
2 g salt

Not That!
Sainsbury's Taste The Difference Steak Au Poivre

Save!
349 calories
16.4 g fat

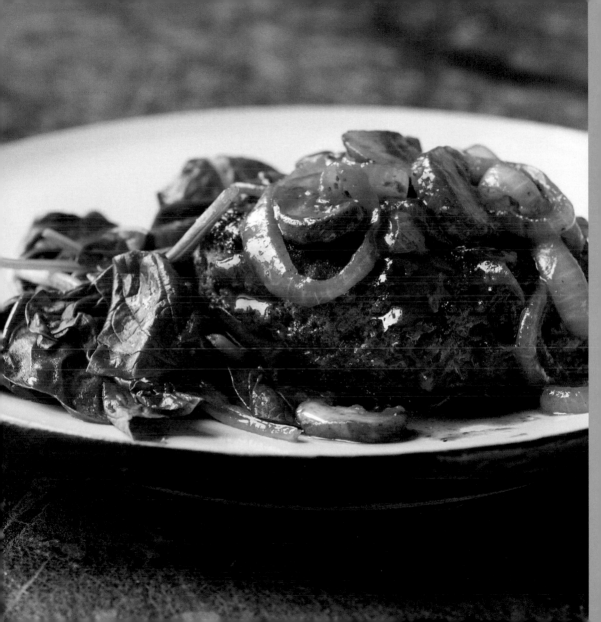

Cook This!

Red Curry Pork Kebab

One of the biggest trends to hit home cooking in the past year is the sudden proliferation of skewers and kebabs. It's a move we fully applaud, since it means that the heavy carbs and fatty sauces that end up on most home plates are being replaced with lean protein and vegetables. These kebabs have plenty of both, all punched up with an addictive Thai curry sauce that you'll find yourself dipping everything in. Pineapple chunks would be a welcome addition here.

You'll Need

120 ml light coconut milk

2 tbsp Thai red curry paste

1 tbsp peanut butter

500 g pork loin, cut into ¾ in pieces

1 red or yellow pepper, chopped into large pieces

1 large red onion, chopped into large pieces

8 wooden skewers, soaked in water for 20 minutes

How To Make It

- Preheat a grill. Combine the coconut milk, curry paste, and peanut butter in a mixing bowl and stir to thoroughly blend. Transfer half to a separate bowl and reserve.

- Thread the pork, pepper, and onion onto the skewers, alternating between the meat and vegetables.

- Use a brush to paint the skewers with some of the remaining curry sauce. When the grill is hot, add the skewers and cook for 3 to 4 minutes per side, basting with a bit more of the sauce as you go.

- The skewers are done when the meat and vegetables are lightly charred and the pork is firm but still slightly yielding to the touch.

- Brush the kebabs with the reserved sauce before serving.

Makes 8 skewers

240 calories
8 g fat
(3.5 g saturated)
0.95 g salt

PER SERVING

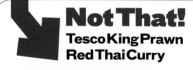

Not That!
Tesco King Prawn Red Thai Curry

460 calories
14.4 g fat
(7.4 g saturated)
2.8 g salt

Save!
220 calories
6.4 g fat

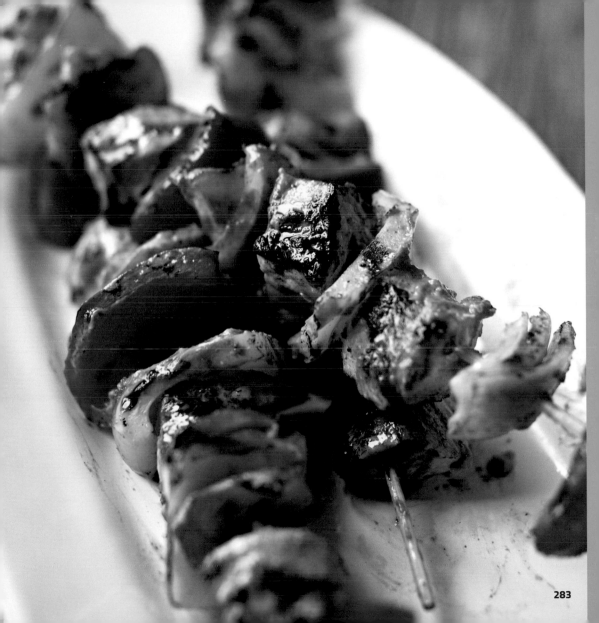

Sea Bass Packet

Why more people don't cook food in packets is one of the culinary world's great mysteries. Not only is it one of the healthiest, easiest ways to cook fish, chicken, and vegetables, but the abundance of flavoursome steam trapped inside the packet means your food will still be delicious, even if you overcook it. Plus, there are no pots or pans to clean—just toss the foil in the trash and move on. Just as easy as a ready meal and far more satisfying.

You'll Need

- **4 sea bass, halibut, or other white fish fillets (150 g each)**
- **8 spears asparagus, ends removed, chopped**
- **110 g shitake mushrooms, stems removed**
- **1 tbsp grated fresh ginger**
- **2 tbsp low-salt soy sauce**
- **2 tbsp mirin (sweetened sake), sake, or sweet white wine**
- **Salt and black pepper to taste**

How To Make It

- Preheat the oven to 200°C/gas mark 6.
- Lay 4 large (18 inch x 12 inch) pieces of foil on the kitchen counter and fold each into thirds. Place a fish fillet in the centre third of each piece, then scatter the asparagus, mushrooms, and ginger over each. Drizzle with the soy sauce and mirin and season with a small pinch of salt (remember, soy sauce already packs plenty of salt) and black pepper. Fold the outer two sections of the foil over the fish, then roll up the ends toward the centre to create fully sealed packets.
- Arrange the packets on a large baking sheet and bake for 15 for 20 minutes, depending on the thickness of the fish fillet. (If the fillets are ½ inch thick or less, it will take closer to 15 minutes; if they are almost a full inch, it will need 20 minutes.) Place each packet directly on a plate and serve.

Serves 4

250 calories
4.5 g fat
(1 g saturated)
1.35 g salt

PER SERVING

Not That!
Waitrose Prawn Cocktail

352 calories
33.6 g fat
(2.6 g saturated)
1.1 g salt

Save!
102 calories
29.1 g fat

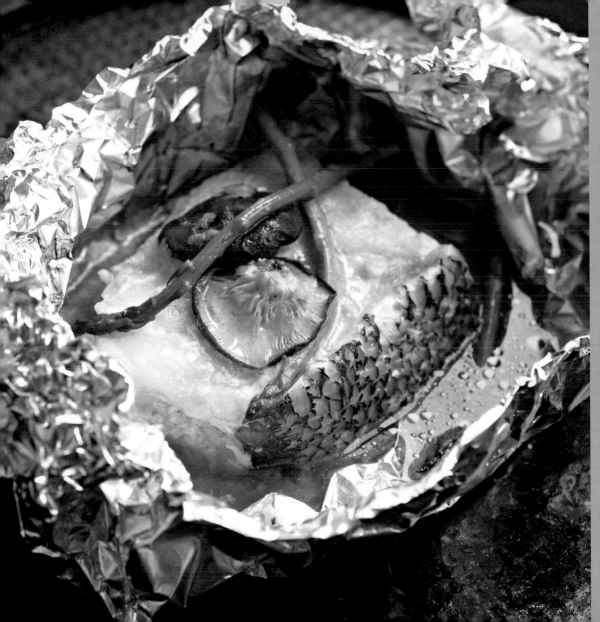

Grilled Steak Taco

We Brits specialise in unhealthy ways to eat steak (such as covering it in pastry or suet). So, next dinner time why not take a leaf out of a typical Mexican cookbook and roll yourself a taco. We've taken the traditional recipe and taken it back to basics, with little more than a fiery marinade (which will boost your metabolism), toasted tortillas, and a scoop of salsa. Oh, and of course, some delicious lean steak.

You'll Need

½ jar of sweet peppers

250 ml orange juice

1 tsp ground cumin

1 tsp chilli powder

2 cloves garlic

500 ml chopped fresh coriander, plus more for garnish

450 g sirloin steak

½ tsp salt

½ tsp pepper

8 corn tortillas

2 tbsp guacamole

Salsa

1 red onion, minced

2 limes, quartered

How To Make It

- Combine the peppers, orange juice, chilli, cumin, garlic, and coriander in a blender and puree. Place the steak and marinate in a resealable plastic bag and refrigerate for 30 minutes or up to 8 hours.

- Remove the steak from the marinade. Season with salt and pepper. Heat the grill, or cast-iron skillet until hot. Cook the steak for 3 to 4 minutes per side (for medium rare).

- Heat the tortillas until warm and pliable. It's best to do this on a hot grill or cast-iron skillet, but at a pinch, wrap the tortillas in a damp paper towel and microwave for 45 seconds.

- Slice the steak across the grain into thin pieces and divide among the tortillas. Top with guacamole, salsa, onion, extra coriander, and a squirt of lime juice.

Serves 4

250 calories
7 g fat
(1.5 g saturated)
1.2 g salt

PER SERVING

425 calories
23 g fat
(12 g saturated)
1.3 g salt

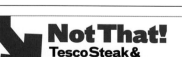

Not That!
Tesco Steak &
Kidney Pudding

Save!
175 calories
16 g fat

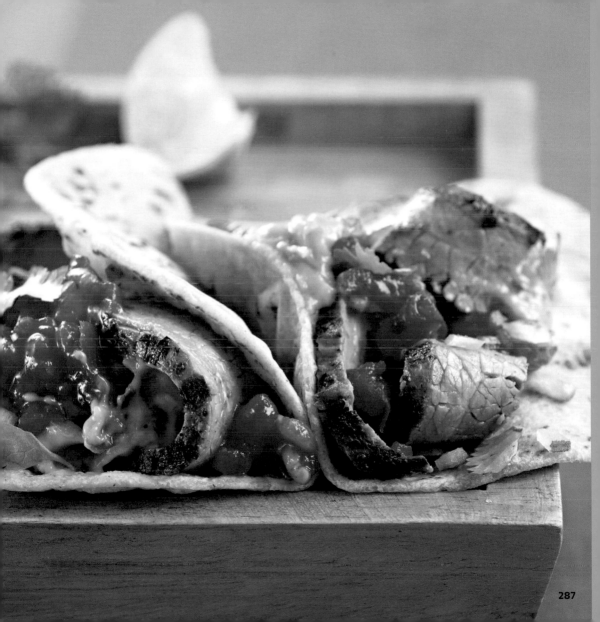

Pork Fillet
Grilled with Pineapple Salsa

Chicken breast may still be king of the UK meat market, but pork fillet (or tenderloin as it's often called) is no less worthy of the crown. Besides being nearly as lean as chicken (it only has 3 grams of fat per 100), pork also boasts an impressive array of nutrients, including more than a third of a day's dose of selenium, a trace mineral shown to be effective in cancer prevention. Another reason to love pork is its ability to stand up to big, gutsy flavours. Here, a heady rub of mustard and chilli powder and a powerful salsa of pineapple and jalapeño help boost the flavour quotient while adding only about 25 calories—plus a tide of first-rate nutrients—to the bottom line.

You'll Need

1 tbsp Dijon or grainy mustard

½ tbsp honey

½ tbsp chilli powder

Salt and black pepper to taste

500 g pork fillet

4 (½ in thick) slices pineapple, core removed

1 red onion, chopped

1 jalapeño pepper, chopped

75 g chopped fresh coriander

Juice of 1 lime

How To Make It

● Preheat the grill. Combine the mustard, honey, chilli powder, and a good sprinkle of salt and pepper and rub all over the pork. Place the pork and pineapple slices on the grill.

● Grill the pineapple for 2 to 3 minutes per side, until lightly charred and softened. Grill the fillet, turning once or twice, for about 10 minutes, until lightly charred and firm (but yielding) to the touch (an internal thermometer should read no more than 70°C). Let the pork rest for at least 5 minutes.

● While the pork rests, chop the pineapple into bite-size pieces. Combine with the onion, jalapeño, coriander, and lime juice. Season with a bit of salt and pepper. Slice the pork and serve with the salsa.

Serves 4

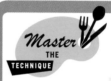

Master **THE** **TECHNIQUE**

Fruit salsa

Nothing impresses more and requires less than a fruit salsa. Start with the same base— a chopped onion jalapeño and some coriander, and the juice of one lime—and then add the fruit of your choice. Mango and papaya are good, but apples, melon, and even strawberries work beautifully as well.

210 calories
4 g fat
(1.5 g saturated)
0.97 g salt

PER SERVING

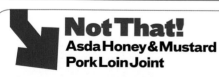

Not That!
Asda Honey & Mustard Pork Loin Joint

353 calories
20.8 g fat
(8.8 g saturated)
0.9 g salt

Save!
143 calories
16.8 g fat

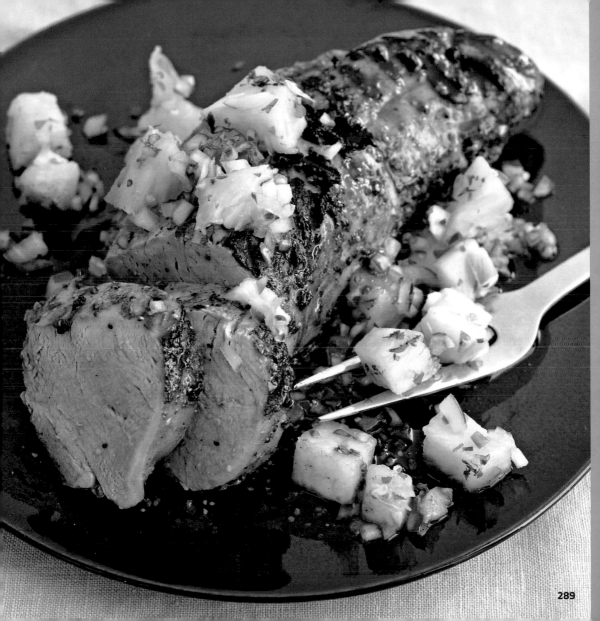

289

Lamb with Tzatziki

Lamb is often third on people's cooking lists after chicken and beef. Too bad, since it is not only jam-packed with flavour and easy to cook, but surprisingly lean when you work with the right cuts. (The notion that lamb is "gamey" doesn't hold true anymore, partially because most lamb is so lean.) Though tzatziki, a Greek-style yogurt sauce, matches perfectly with a charred lamb chop, it also can—and should—be applied to grilled chicken, pork, and fish on a frequent basis.

You'll Need

1 cucumber, peeled, halved, and seeded

250 ml Greek-style yogurt

Juice of 1 lemon

2 tbsp olive oil

2 cloves garlic, finely minced

2 tsp minced fresh dill

Salt and black pepper to taste

4 loin or shoulder lamb chops (about 100 g each)

How To Make It

● Preheat a grill. Grate the cucumber with a cheese grater, then use your hands to wring out all the excess water. Combine the cucumber with the yogurt, lemon juice, half the olive oil, garlic, dill, and a good pinch of salt and pepper. This is your tzatziki. Set it aside.

● Rub the lamb with the remaining olive oil, then season all over with salt and pepper. Grill, turning once, until a meat thermometer inserted into the deepest part of a chop reads 60°C, 10 to 12 minutes, depending on the thickness of the cut. Serve with the tzatziki.

Serves 4

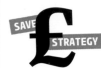

260 calories
15 g fat
(4 g saturated)
0.97 g salt

PER SERVING

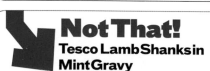

Not That!
Tesco Lamb Shanks in Mint Gravy

607 calories
26.3 g fat
(10.5 g saturated)
2.8 g salt

Save!
347 calories
11.3 g fat

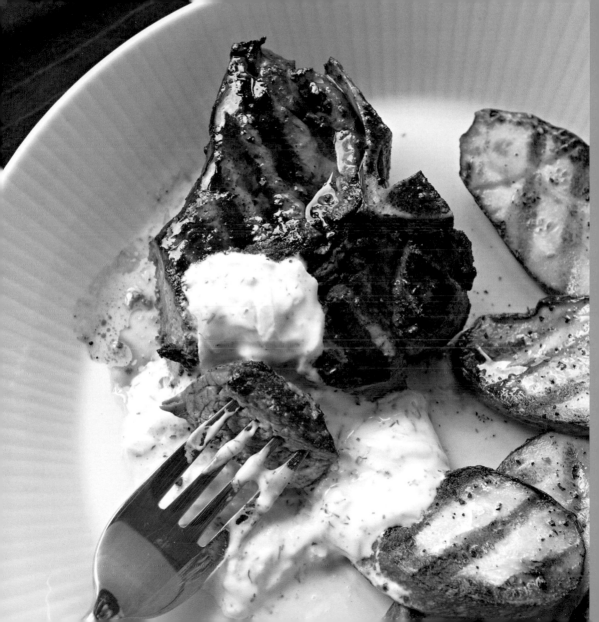

Pesto-Grilled Swordfish

No fridge should be without a jar of pesto. It pairs perfectly with pasta, of course, but also works as an excellent sandwich spread, salad dressing enhancer, and instant marinade. This recipe takes the latter tack, slathering meaty swordfish steaks in pesto before grilling, then topping them with quick-sautéed tomatoes. The burst of sweetness from the tomatoes joins forces with the garlicky punch of the pesto, making for a dish that tastes every bit the creation of a restaurant chef.

You'll Need

- **2 tbsp pesto**
- **4 swordfish steaks (120 g each)**
- **1 tbsp olive oil**
- **2 cloves garlic, peeled and lightly crushed**
- **300 g cherry tomatoes**
- **Salt and black pepper to taste**

How To Make It

- Spread the pesto all over the swordfish steaks, cover, and marinate in the fridge for 30 minutes.
- While the fish marinates, heat the olive oil in a frying pan over medium heat. Add the garlic and cook for a minute or two, until lightly browned. Add the tomatoes and fry until the skins are lightly blistered and about to pop, about 5 minutes. Season with salt and pepper.
- Preheat a grill or grill pan. Season the fish all over with salt and pepper. When the grill is hot, cook the swordfish for 4 to 5 minutes per side, until the fish is cooked all the way through and the flesh flakes with gentle pressure. Reheat the tomatoes and top each steak with a scoop.

Serves 4

Upgrade

NUTRITIONAL

Greater grains

UK eating traditions dictate that every home-cooked meal comes with a starch, which usually means potatoes or rice, neither of which add much to a meal other than empty carbs. But a new class of global grains is now available that can cut calories and boost nutrition. quinoa is one of the best, but also try amaranth, couscous, and farro. All are excellent high-fibre rice and potato alternatives.

250 calories
13 g fat
(3 g saturated)
0.97 g salt

PER SERVING

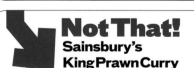

Not That!
Sainsbury's King Prawn Curry

422 calories
11 g fat
(5.8 g saturated)
1.9 g salt

Save!
172 calories
2 g fat

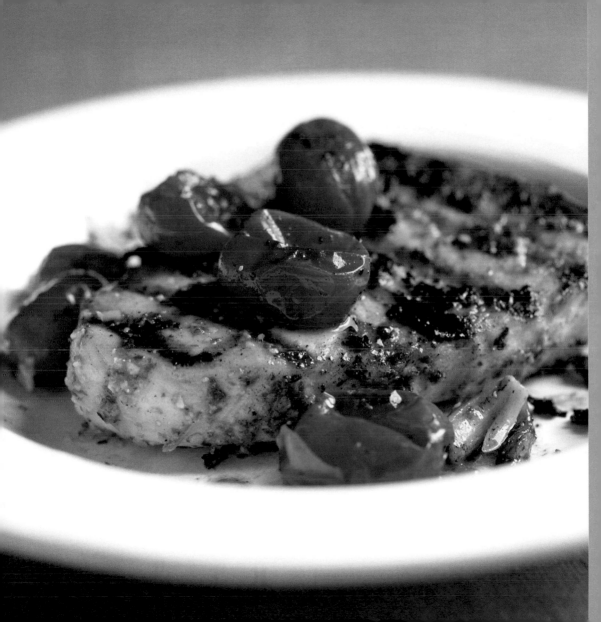

Molten Chocolate Cake

The idea of baking and frosting a multi-tiered chocolate cake is daunting for most, but these little self-contained parcels of joy are the lazy man's cake, the type of dessert that makes a non-baker feel like a patisserie king when they emerge from the oven, pregnant with a tide of melted chocolate. Crack the middle and watch the flood of lava flow freely onto your plate—and eventually into your eagerly awaiting mouth. Did we mention these have only 360 calories?

You'll Need

- **140 g dark chocolate (at least 60% cacao), plus 4 chunks for the cake centres**
- **2 tbsp butter**
- **2 eggs**
- **2 egg yolks**
- **50 g sugar**
- **Pinch of salt**
- **2 tbsp flour**
- **1 tsp vanilla extract**
- **½ tbsp instant coffee or espresso (optional)**

How To Make It

- Preheat the oven to 220°C/gas mark 7. Lightly butter four ramekins or espresso cups.
- Bring a few cups of water to a boil in a medium saucepan over low heat. Place a glass mixing bowl over the pan (but not touching the water) and add the chocolate and butter. Cook, stirring occasionally, until both the chocolate and butter have fully melted. Keep warm.
- Use an electric mixer to beat the eggs, egg yolks, sugar, and salt until pale yellow and thick, about 5 minutes. Stir in the melted chocolate mixture, the flour, vanilla, and instant coffee if using.
- Pour the mixture into the prepared ramekins. Stick one good chunk of chocolate in the centre of each ramekin. Bake the cakes on the centre rack for 8 to 10 minutes, until the exterior is just set (the centre should still be mostly liquid). The cakes can be eaten straight from the ramekins, but it's more dramatic to slide them on to plates (after letting them rest for a minute or two), where the molten chocolate can flow freely.

Makes 4 servings

360 calories
26 g fat
(13 g saturated)
trace salt

PER SERVING

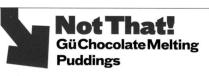

Not That!
Gü Chocolate Melting Puddings

421 calories
27.4 g fat
(16.3 g saturated)
trace salt

Save!
61 calories
3.3 g sat fat

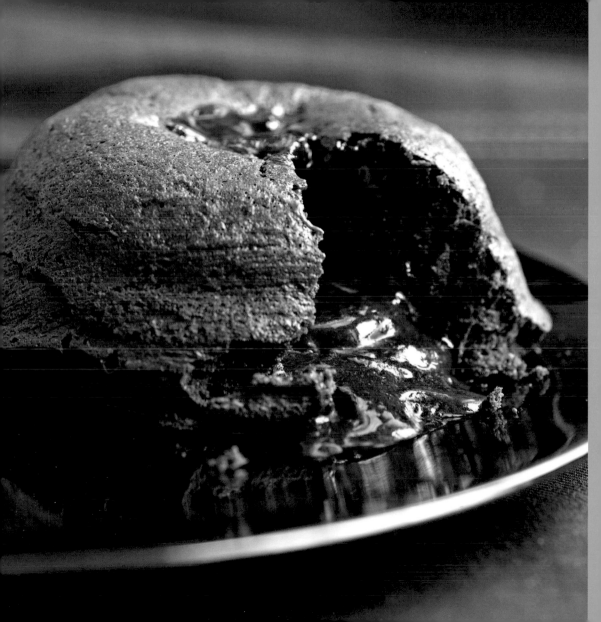

Sundae with Grilled Pineapple & Rum Sauce

The banana may be the sundae fruit vessel of choice, but the standard split formula—one banana, three scoops ice cream—is a disastrous recipe for the discerning eater. Pineapple, on the other hand, holds one good scoop of ice cream perfectly, and its kick of sweetness and acidity—which is only intensified when it's grilled—matches nicely with the creamy vanilla. Add a swirl of rum sauce and some toasted coconut and it's like having a piña colada, minus the hangover.

You'll Need

- **4 (½ in thick) slices fresh pineapple, core removed**
- **1 tbsp butter**
- **2 tbsp brown sugar**
- **2 tbsp dark rum**
- **1 tsp vanilla extract**
- **500 ml vanilla ice cream**
- **2 tbsp shredded sweetened coconut**

How To Make It

- The first stage of this recipe (toasting the coconut) is optional but highly recommended, as it will help not only the flavour, but the texture of the dish, too. To toast, spread your shredded coconut on a baking tray and put it in a pre-heated oven at 180°C/gas mark 4 for 12 minutes, until golden brown. Skip this if you're pushed for time.
- Heat a griddle pan, or large frying pan over medium heat (using a small knob of butter in the frying pan). Cook the pineapple rings for 3 to 4 minutes per side, until caramelised all over. Then take them off the heat and set aside.
- Cook the butter, brown sugar, rum, and vanilla in a saucepan over low heat, stirring occasionally, until the sugar fully melts and the sauce is a uniform dark brown. Keep warm.
- Place one slice of pineapple on each of 4 small plates. Top with a scoop of ice cream, drizzle on the rum sauce, then finish with the toasted coconut.

Serves 4

290 calories
11 g fat
(7 g saturated)
35 g sugar

PER SERVING

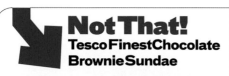

Not That!
Tesco Finest Chocolate Brownie Sundae

540 calories
27 g fat
(16.8 g saturated)
52 g sugar

Save!
250 calories
17 g sugar

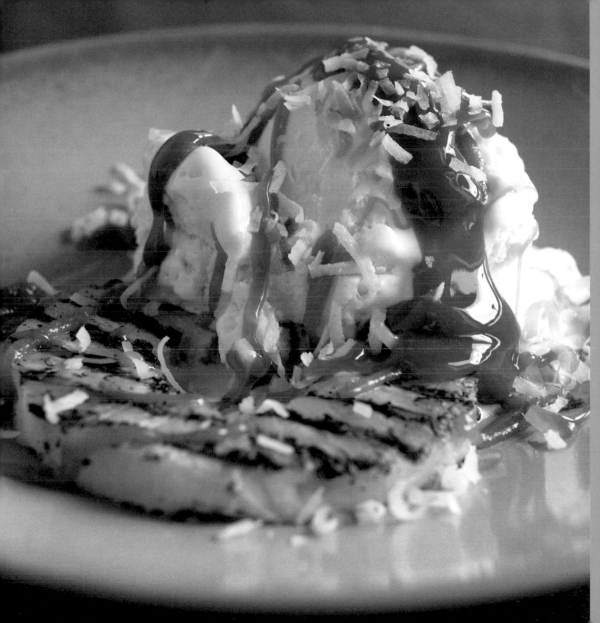

Chapter

8

FOR KIDS

Being a great parent

has—let's face it—always been hard work. Pity poor Adam and Eve, trying to work out the whole parenting thing without a guidebook. (Eve: "Should we be concerned about Cain picking on his brother?" Adam: "Nah, they're fine. Hand me an apple.") Or how about the mythical Oedipus, who ended up killing his dad and marrying his mum? (And you thought your children feeding the dog their spinach was a problem...)

But while headaches, backaches, and wallet aches have always been part of the penalty we pay for having kids, it seems as though parenting has become even more complicated in recent years. Technology deserves its fair share of the blame: Facebook, texting, and the like have given our progeny plenty of ways to get around the rules. But the technology that's complicating our lives as parents is a different kind of science entirely.

FOOD SCIENCE

The foods our children are eating today are very different from the foods we ate at their age. The foods in today's supermarkets and on restaurant kids' menus come not from the great green earth, but from the minds of marketers. And they're assembled not in warm, welcoming kitchens, but in cold, bright science labs—complete with nutritional labels that read more like the contents of a chemistry set.

Consider if you will, the humble Coco Pop. A small puff of delight that has been feeding children a mildly indulgent breakfast since 1958. It seems to be little more than chocolate toasted rice, right? Well although the Coco Pops you or I grew up with may have been a tad sugary, it was a pretty simple recipe. But then things got complicated. Because now we have not only Kellogg's Coco Pops but also Coco Pops Choc'n'Roll, Coco Rocks, Moon & Stars and Coco Pops cereal bars.

Which of these variations are good for your kids? Which are not?

It's hard to tell. Is the "potassium chloride" in the Choc'n'Roll something you should feed your kids? What about the 5 grams of fat in a serving of the Coco Rocks, or the glucose syrup, the cocoa mass, and oh yes the actual sugar (which is listed three times)? In fact, these breakfast concoctions are a great example of how today's food companies are taking foods and messing around with a complex combination of confusing, ambiguous ingredients.

The result of all this fiddling about with our food supply is easy to see all around us: Children are getting fatter. And with that fat comes

What Our Children Need Each Day

	1–3 YEARS	4–8 YEARS	9–13 YEARS	14–18 YEARS
CALORIES	1,000–1,400	1,400–1,600	1,800–2,200 (BOY)	2,200–2,400 (BOY)
			1,600–2,200 (GIRL)	2,000 (GIRL)
FAT (g)	33–54	39–62	62–85	61–95 (B) 55–78 (G)
SATURATED FAT (g)	<12–16	<16–18	<20–24 (B) <18–22 (G)	<24–27 (B) <22 (G)
SODIUM (mg)	1,000–1,500	1,200–1,900	1,500–2,200	1,500–2,300
CARBS (g)	130	130	130	130
FIBRE (g)	19	25	31 (B) 26 (G)	38 (B) 26 (G)
PROTEIN (g)	13	19	31 (B) 26 (G)	52 (B) 46 (G)

more than just jokes about your "junk-food junkies" and school shirts straining at the buttons. Being overweight as a child is a serious health problem. Consider this:

Ten years ago, type 2 diabetes was known as "adult-onset diabetes" because it took several decades of overeating to get your body to the point where it was at risk. But we have so hyperinflated the calories in our foods that even children as young as four are now developing this disease. And it's not a pretty disease: Among its complications are blindness, heart attacks, strokes and sexual dysfunction. There are now roughly 2.8 million people in the UK living with diabetes.

Yet much of the food on offer as "for kids" in UK restaurants and supermarkets is a practical invitation to diabetes and other health complications—from heart disease to cancer to high blood pressure to asthma—later in life.

That's why we've included this chapter. We've uncovered the real truth about what the UK is feeding its children. And the great news is this: You can have a major impact on your children's health and future, simply by making a few smart choices.

The power is in your hands.

Eat This Pyramid

There are two ways children learn about nutrition in schools. One is the food plate (now adopted by the FSA—see page 315 for more on this). The other is the classic 'food pyramid', which leaves a lot to be desired in terms of specifics. For example a serving of white rice counts the same towards six daily servings of grains as a serving of quinoa—despite the fact that one is packed with fibre, healthy fats and essential amino acids (quinoa) and the other is a nutritional black hole (rice). Likewise, all meats are lumped into the same category despite the vast difference between omega-rich fish and a fatty beef burger. Here we've created our own version of the pyramid, which gives a much more accurate breakdown of what to eat, and what not to. Turn to page 308 for further detail on fruit and veg and, more specifically, how eating different colours is an excellent and easy-to-understand way to ensure your children stay well-nourished.

FATS AND OILS (USE SPARINGLY)

Eat This
Healthy fats: olive oil; canola oil; monounsaturated fats from nuts, avocado and salmon

NotThat!
Unhealthy fats: margarine; lard; salted butter; palm oil; anything with partially hydrogenated oil

DAIRY (2 OR 3 SERVINGS)

Eat This
Semi-skimmed milk; cottage cheese; plain yogurt or fromage frais sweetened with fresh fruit

NotThat!
Chocolate milk; ice cream; melted cheese; yogurts with a high sugar content

MEAT, FISH, EGGS, NUTS AND BEANS (2 OR 3 SERVINGS)

Eat This
Grilled chicken breast; roast pork tenderloin; sirloin steak; oily fish; boiled or poached eggs; kidney beans; chickpeas; almonds; unsweetened nut butters

NotThat!
Chicken nuggets; fried chicken; cheeseburgers; deep-fried battered cod; processed meats; salted nuts or peanut butter with added sugar

VEGETABLES (5 SERVINGS)

Eat This
Sautéed spinach; steamed broccoli; romaine or mixed green salads; roasted mushrooms; grilled pepper and onion skewers; baby carrots; homemade tomato sauce

NotThat!
Chips; crisps; onion rings or other battered vegetables; veg in cheese or creamy sauces

FRUIT (3 SERVINGS)

Eat This
Sliced apples or pears; berries; grapes; pure fruit smoothies; stone fruit such as peaches, plums and apricots

NotThat!
More than one glass of juice a day; more than a handful of dried fruit a day; smoothies made with sugar; canned fruit in syrup

GRAINS (6 SERVINGS)

Eat This
Brown rice; wholemeal bread; quinoa; wholemeal pasta; barley; oatmeal;

NotThat!
White rice; white bread; muffins; tortillas; pancakes; waffles; heavily sweetened cereal

303

8 Rules of Kids' Nutrition

Rule #1

NEVER SKIP BREAKFAST. EVER

Yes, mornings are crazy. But they're also our best hope at regaining our nutritional sanity. A 2005 study combined the results of 47 other studies that examined the impact of starting the day with a healthy breakfast. Here's what they found.

Children skipped breakfast more than any other meal. Skipping is more prevalent in girls, older children, and in adolescents.

People who skip breakfast are more likely to take up smoking or drinking, less likely to exercise, and more likely to follow fad diets or express concerns about body weight. Common reasons cited for skipping were lack of time, lack of hunger, or dieting. Bad news. True, it would seem to make sense that skipping breakfast means eating fewer calories, which means weighing less. But it doesn't work that way.

People who eat breakfast tend to have higher total calorie intakes throughout the day, but they also get significantly more fibre, calcium, and other micronutrients than skippers do. Breakfast eaters also tended to consume less fizzy drinks and chips and more fruits, vegetables, and milk.

Breakfast eaters were 30 percent less likely to be overweight or obese. (Think about that—kids who eat breakfast eat more food, but still weigh less!)

Rule #2

SNACK WITH PURPOSE

There's a big difference between mindless munching and strategic snacking. Snacking with purpose means reinforcing good habits, keeping your metabolic rate high, and filling the gaps between meals with the nutrients your body craves. Combat crisp binges by sending your child off to school with healthy snacks that you'll both feel good about: Crackers and peanut butter; a pot of yogurt; a handful of dried apricots or raisins; some carrot sticks and a pot of hummus.

Rule #3
WATCH SCHOOL DINNERS

Speaking of school dinners, you'd think now that Jamie Oliver has fought the system it would be safe to send your kids to school with a pocket full of change to spend as they see fit in the canteen.

Jamie's revolution brought in new guidelines in 2008 and 2009 which included a ban on sweets and other food nasties sold in schools, along with a guarantee that all children would be provided with at least two portions of fruit and vegetables each and every day. And according to the latest figures the number of pupils opting for school meals is on the increase: more than two-fifths of primary school children and a third of secondary school pupils.

But, with a quarter of under-10s obese (the highest rate of childhood obesity in Europe) and a third of teenagers, if you're not packing their lunch then you do need to check what they're eating—a school meal accounts for a third of your child's daily intake. And who's to say they aren't spending some of their dinner money at the local sweet shop?

Rule #4
BEWARE OF PORTION DISTORTION

In the 20 year period between 1977 and 1996, salty snack portions increased by 93 calories, and soft drink portions increased by 49 calories. So when you give your kid an individual bag of crisps and a can of fizzy drink—the same snack you might have enjoyed when you were 10 years old—they're ingesting 142 more calories than you did. Feeding them that just twice a week means they could gain up to 4 pounds a year. And snack portions aren't the only things on the up. Since 1977, burgers have increased by 97 calories and a portion of chips by 68 calories, according to a US analysis of the Nation-wide Food Consumption Survey. One easy way to short-circuit this growing trend? *Buy smaller bowls and cups.* A recent study at the Children's Nutrition Research Center in Houston, Texas, shows that five- and six-year-old children will consume a third more calories when presented with a larger portion. The findings are based on a sample of 53 children who were served either 250- or 500-gram portions of macaroni cheese.

Rule #5
DRINK RESPONSIBLY

Too many of us keep in mind the adage "watch what you eat," while forgetting another serious threat to our health: We don't watch what we drink. One important strategy is to keep cold, filtered water in a jug in the fridge. You might even want to keep some cut-up limes, oranges or lemons nearby for your children to flavour their own water with. A British study showed that in classrooms with limited access to water, only 29 percent of students met their daily needs; free access to water led to a much higher daily intake of H_2O.

Be extra careful about the juice you purchase. Too many "juices" are little more than sugar water masquerading as the real thing. Ocean Spray Cranberry and Raspberry, for instance, has just 20 percent real fruit juice. The other 80 percent? Sugar and water. Make sure the juice you buy says "100 percent fruit juice" on the label, and try to choose one made from a single fruit, not a mix of high-sugar fruits such as white grapes, which are commonly used in fruit juice blends. And after you find the perfect juice, limit kids to one 250ml glass a day. If they want more, hand them a glass of water and a piece of fruit.

Rule #6
EAT MORE WHOLE FOODS AND FEWER SCIENCE EXPERIMENTS

Here's a rule of healthy eating that will serve you well when picking out foods for your family in the future: the shorter the ingredients list, the healthier the food. (One of the worst foods ever found in the US version of this book was the Baskin-Robbins Heath Shake, with an incredible 73 ingredients, along with a whopping 2,310 calories and more than 3 days' worth of saturated fat. What happened to the idea that a milk shake was, um, milk, and ice cream? Let's just be grateful that Baskin-Robbins finally pulled this monstrosity from its menus before it hit the shores of the UK.)

Rule #7
SET THE TABLE

Children in families with structured mealtimes exhibit healthier eating habits. Among teenage girls, those whose families ate together only once or twice per week were more than twice as likely to exhibit weight control issues, compared with those who ate together three or four times per week.

Of course, the notion of a 6pm dinnertime "and then everyone into their PJs" is a quaint one, but hardly realistic in a society where children have such highly scheduled social lives that the delineation between "parent" and "chauffeur" is sometimes difficult to parse. While we can't always bring the family together, we can make some positive steps in that direction. One way busy families can do this is to keep Sunday night dinner sacred—no social plans, no school projects, no extra work brought home from the office. Even sticking to this family ritual just one day a week gives parents the opportunity to point out what is and isn't healthy at the dinner table.

Another smart move: Get your children involved in cooking. Make a game of trying to pack the healthiest ingredients into your meals. One Texas study showed that children can be encouraged to eat more fruits and vegetables by

giving them goals and allowing them to help prepare their own meals. You could even buy your children their own aprons and cutting boards, and let them peel carrots and stir sauces. If at the end of the day they've done their duties as diligent sous chefs, then reward them with that age-old kitchen treasure: A few licks of the cake mix off the back of the spoon.

Rule #8
BEWARE OF RESTAURANTS

Not only should you have one eye on the nutritional information of your own meal, but the other should be firmly on the children's choice. Don't assume that because it is marked as a children's meal on the menu that it will be a smaller portion and therefore a healthy option.

Take JD Wetherspoon's children's breakfast for example (that's if you take your children to breakfast in the pub), which is complete with sausage, bacon, baked beans, a fried egg and a hash brown. It is also complete with 630 calories, 37 grams of fat, over 10 grams of saturated fat and a whopping 4.8 grams of salt. They say, "suitable for children under 10." We disagree.

Eat the Rainbow!

Let's not pretend that getting kids to eat what's good for them isn't sometimes a struggle. "A lot of parents tell me, 'My kids don't like healthy foods,'" says David Katz, an associate clinical professor of epidemiology and public health at Yale Medical School. "'Fussy' is not an excuse. You never hear a parent say, 'My child doesn't like to look both ways before he crosses the street.' They tell him to do it. More kids today will die of complications from bad foods they eat than will die from tobacco, drugs, and alcohol."

So how do you teach the basics of nutrition to a seven-year-old? Even we grown-ups have trouble understanding how many calories we're supposed to take in each day, which vitamins and minerals we need more of, and which of the complicated chemical ingredients flooding our food system we need to avoid.

Well, here's a simple trick: Just teach your kids to eat as many different colours as they can. And no, we're not talking about red, green, and purple Skittles. We're talking about eating as much of a mix of fruits and veg as possible. That's because the colours represented in foods are indicators of nutritional value—and different colours mean different vitamins and minerals.

Not everything on this list is going to appeal to your child. But there's enough variation here that he or she can squeeze one food from each category into a day's eating. For a fun project, make a multicolour checklist and have your child check off each colour as he or she eats it throughout the day.

Or do what our parents did and sell them on the child-friendly benefits trapped inside of spinach, carrots, and the like. Each group of produce offers seriously cool "superpowers" that appeal to kids' deepest desires to dominate science tests and football games alike. Feel free to sell these as hard as you want. Hey, even if it didn't end up making you as strong as Popeye, you still ate your spinach, didn't you?

Red

Rosy-hued fruit and veg contain the antioxidant lycopene, which has a cache of health benefits, including protecting the skin from sun damage and decreasing the risk of heart disease and certain forms of cancer. Lycopene is most strongly concentrated in the reddest of all red fruits: the tomato. What is surprising, though, is that cooked and processed tomatoes have higher concentrations of lycopene, so don't shy away from the salsa or marinara sauce.

SUPERPOWER Superman speed. Lycopene-rich foods have been shown to decrease symptoms of wheezing, asthma and shortness of breath in people when they exercise.

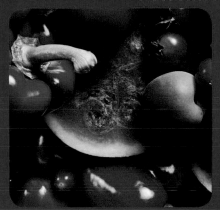

TOMATOES
This queen of lycopene is also packed with anti-oxidant-rich vita-mins A and C, as well as vitamin K, which is vital for maintaining healthy bones. Canned and cooked tomatoes have been shown to contain more lycopene than fresh, so go crazy with the salsa and marinara sauce. When possible, buy organic: USDA researchers found that organic ketchup has three times the lycopene as normal ketchup.

RED PEPPERS
The red ones pack twice the vitamin C and nine times the vitamin A as their green relatives. They've been shown to aid in the fight against every-thing from asthma to cancer. Slice them up raw and serve with some hummus for an after-school snack, or buy a jar of pre-roasted peppers and puree them into a soup. (It tastes just like tomato soup.)

GUAVA
Like most lycopene vessels, guava is packed with vitamins A and C. It also contains heart-healthy omega-3 fatty acids and belly-filling fibre. Get your hands on these in the fresh produce aisles of larger supermarkets or simply keep a bottle of guava nectar in the fridge.

WATERMELON
This summertime favorite is also a big provider of vitamins A and C, which help to neutralise cancer-causing free radicals. Spike a fruit salad with big chunks of watermelon; blend it with yogurt, ice and juice for a refreshing smoothie; or just cut one up on a hot day after you've fired up the barbecue.

PINK GRAPEFRUIT
This contains one of the highest concentrations of antioxidants in the fruit bowl. Mix segments into yogurt and cereal in the morning for breakfast, slip them into salads, or just swap the orange juice for the occasional glass of ruby red grapefruit.

Orange

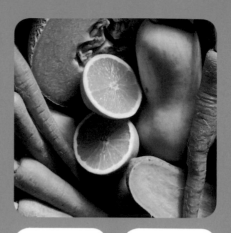

Beta-carotene is the nutrient responsible for dramatic oranges in fruit and veg. But the conspicuous hue of this carotenoid does more than just attract your attention; once inside your body, it is converted into vitamin A, a powerful antioxidant that contributes to immune health and helps fight off cell-damaging free radicals.

SUPERPOWER Orange foods give you night vision! That's because vitamin A is vital for creating the pigment in the retina responsible for vision in low-light situations. Just think of the benefits: It'll help them beat their friends at hide-and-seek or spy on their brothers and sisters.

SWEET POTATOES

The best thing about sweet potatoes, outside of the beta-carotene, is that they're loaded with fibre. That means they have a gentler effect on blood sugar levels than regular potatoes. Substitute baked sweet potatoes for jacket potatoes, mash them up as normal, or make chips out of them by tossing spears with olive oil and roasting for 30 minutes.

ORANGES

This vaunted vitamin C monster has a cadre of critical phytonutrients known to lower blood pressure and contain strong anti-inflammatory properties. Juice is fine, but the real fruit is even better. The secret, though, is that the orange's most powerful healing properties are found in the peel; use a zester to grate the peel over bowls of yogurt, salads, or directly into smoothies.

BUTTERNUT SQUASH

A true nutritional powerhouse, winter squash is a great source of various vitamins, including a host of B vitamins, folate, manganese, and fibre. What does that all mean? It means feed it to your child—and lots of it! The best way is t o cut the squash into 1-inch wedges and bake for 40 minutes, until they're soft and caramelised.

MELONS

The surge of vitamin A is important not just for your eyes, but also for healthy lungs, and the mega-dose of vitamin C helps white blood cells ward off infection. Sliced cantaloupe and yogurt makes a killer breakfast, or combine the two in a blender with a touch of honey and lemon, and puree into a soup. It makes a great low-calorie dessert.

CARROTS

The snack of choice for Bugs Bunny happens to be the richest carotene source of all. Raw baby carrots are perfect for dipping or snacking on, of course, but also try shredding carrots into a salad or marinara for a hint of natural sweetness, or roasting them slowly in the oven with olive oil and a pinch of salt.

Yellow

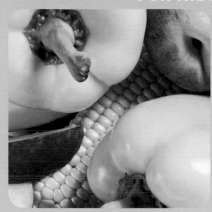

Yellow foods are rich in carotenoid beta-cryptoxanthin and are a good source of vitamin A. Studies show it decreases the likelihood of such diseases as lung cancer and arthritis, but since youngsters have more important things to worry about, you're better off selling these foods on the superpowers they bestow.

SUPERPOWER Yellow foods make you jump higher and play better! Research shows beta-cryptoxanthin helps decrease inflammation in the joints, ensuring a springy steps. Studies also show it may improve the functioning of the respiratory system, making showing up their friends in the pool or on the pitch that much easier.

BANANAS
Bananas are loaded with potassium, which will help your kids grow strong, durable bones. They also contain prebiotics, which makes it easier for eaters to absorb all kinds of nutrients. Shopping tip: Not all bananas are equally rich in carotenoids. Search for those with a deeper gold to their peels.

YELLOW PEPPERS
These peppers are vitamin C treasure troves, providing over twice the amount you'd get from an orange. Their sweet, mellow flavor is perfect for kids, making them an easy addition to stir-fries and sandwiches, and they're great cooked under the grill and served as a side to chicken.

PINEAPPLES
This fruit might be high on the list of carotenoid-containing fruits, but it has other benefits, as well—notably an abundance of bromelain, which aids digestion. Skewer chunks and cook them under a hot grill for a killer dessert.

SWEET CORN
This summer barbecue side-dish is loaded with thiamin, which plays a central role in energy production and cognitive function. Boost their brains and energy levels by carefully removing the kernels from the cob with a knife and sautéing with a bit of olive oil. Eat as it is, or sprinkle the toasty corn niblets on top of soups and salads.

YELLOW SQUASH
With generous doses of fibre, manganese, magnesium and folate, these squashes prove to be a serious nutritional player. Drizzle grilled slices with a bit of pesto.

Green

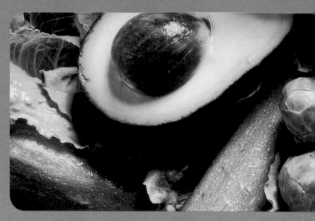

Not just vitamin vessels capable of strengthening bones, muscles and brains, green foods are also some of the most abundant sources of lutein and zeaxanthin—an antioxidant tag team that promotes healthy vision.

SUPERPOWER Green foods give you sharp vision and superhuman healing abilities! Green fruits and vegetables get their colour from chlorophyll, which plays an important role in stimulating the growth of new tissue and hindering the growth of bacteria. It can actually speed healing time by 25 percent.

AVOCADOS
This creamy fruit is bursting with monounsaturated fats, the kind that are proven to be great for your heart. Tossing avocado slices into sandwiches and soups is one way to add some healthy fat, but your best bet for slipping them into your child's diet is to mash 'em up with garlic, onion, and lemon juice for a tasty homemade guacamole.

ASPARAGUS
These potent spears contain a special kind of carbohydrate called inulin, which promotes the growth of healthy bacteria in our large intestines, forcing out the more mischievous kind. Wrap spears in thin slices of ham and bake at about 200°C/gas mark 6 until the ham turns crispy.

ROMAINE LETTUCE
Whereas the ubiquitous iceberg has nary a nutrient to its name, romaine is bursting at the leaves with everything from bone-strengthening vitamin K to folic acid, which is essential to cardiovascular health. Other good, nutrient-dense lettuces for salads and sandwiches include red leaf, and rocket.

BRUSSELS SPROUTS
One of the strongest natural cancer-fighters on the planet, brussels sprouts too often get a bad rap for being boring. Combat the boredom by roasting at around 230°C/gas mark 8 until crispy and caramelised, then tossing them with sliced almonds and golden raisins.

SPINACH
This is one of your best sources of folate, which keeps your body in good supply of oxygen-carrying red blood cells. If your children aren't ready to eat it from the can like Popeye, try frying it in olive oil until fully wilted, then scrambling it into eggs or mixing it into pasta.

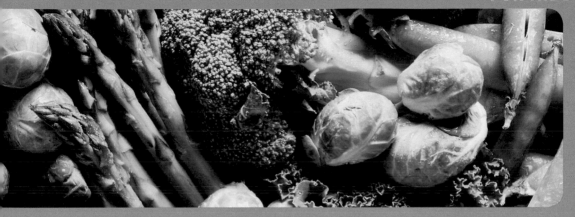

KALE
Aside from containing nearly two weeks' worth of bone strengthening vitamin K, each serving of these deep green leaves has fewer than 40 calories and nearly 10 percent of your RDA of calcium. Fry in olive oil until wilted, then add raisins and toasted pine nuts.

BROCCOLI
These little trees have two days' worth of vitamins C and K in each serving. Top a baked potato with a few steamed florets and a bit of grated cheese, or serve chopped-up pieces alongside a tub of hummus and see if the dip doesn't get the children interested.

KIWIS
Not only do kiwis pack more vitamin C than oranges, they also lay claim to a bulky portfolio of polyphoneols and carotenoids, some of which may have protective effects on our respiratory health. An Italian study found that children who consumed more kiwis had fewer problems with shortness of breath, wheezing, and coughing. Try layering slices of kiwi with yogurt for a healthy dessert.

COURGETTES
A dense and diverse source of nutrients, this summer squash comes with everything from omega-3s to copper. Toss sautéed courgette with a drizzle of balsamic vinegar, or add grated courgette to your favourite bread or cake recipe.

PEAS
Beyond the abundance of vitamins and minerals, a cup of peas contains more than a third of your child's daily fibre intake—more than many wholemeal breads. Add frozen peas to a pasta sauce at the last second, or puree them with garlic and olive oil for a simple, sweet dip.

Blue
and Purple

Blue and purple foods get their colours from flavonoids called anthocyanins. They improve cardiovascular health and prevent short-term memory loss. A study at Tufts University also found that blueberries may make brain cells respond better to incoming messages and might even spur the growth of new nerve cells, giving new meaning to "smart eating."

SUPERPOWER You'll be top of the class!

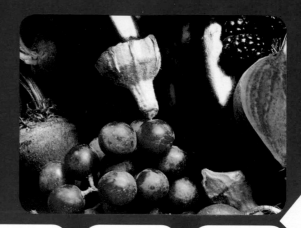

AUBERGINES
A pigment called nasunin is concentrated in the peel of the aubergine, and studies have shown that it has powerful disease-fighting properties. For a child-friendly dinner, try layering half-inch-thick slices of aubergine with tomato sauce and mozzarella cheese and baking for 25 minutes.

RADISHES
Nutritional benefits vary among the many varieties of radishes, but they all share an abundance of vitamin C and a tendency to facilitate the digestive process. Try thinly sliced radishes on a bagel with low-fat cream cheese and black pepper.

GRAPES
Despite their high-fat diets, the French are protected from heart disease by their mass consumption of grapes and wine. Look for a deeper shade of purple—that indicates a high flavonoid concentration. Try freezing grapes in the summer for a cool, healthy treat—or use them frozen as sweet ice cubes.

BEETROOT
This sweet vegetable gets most of its colour from a cancer-fighting pigment called betacyanin. The edible root is replete with fibre, potassium, and manganese. Toss roasted beetroot chunks with toasted walnuts and orange segments, or grate it raw into salads.

BLACKBERRIES
One cup of berries contains 5 percent of your child's daily folate and half the day's vitamin C. Try pureeing blackberries, then combining them with olive oil and balsamic vinegar for a super healthy salad dressing.

Eat This Plate, Not That One!

Simplicity is elegant. It's the case in nutrition as it is in design. The Food Standards Authority must have recognised this truth when it introduced the NHS-sanctioned Eatwell Plate in 2007: divided into colour-coded sections, with each representing the proportion of each food group we should be eating as part of our daily meals. The Eatwell Plate served as a welcome replacement for the somewhat confusing 'Balance of Good Health', with vague labels such as "meat alternatives" ditched in favour of helpful descriptions ("eggs, beans and other sources of protein").

But still, the growing need for clear parental guidance is starkly evident: Almost one in four children is already overweight by the time they start primary school, and with 80% of kids forgoing their five-a-day in favour of artery-clogging, energy-jolting junk foods, our childhood obesity rates are fast catching up with the table-toppers across the pond.

We do applaud the FSA's attempts to provide some clarity, but even the Eatwell Plate leaves room for error. So in the name of *true* simplicity, we've broken down the best and worst options for each food group.

Eat This

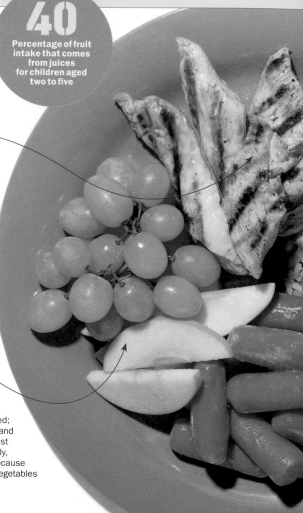

40
Percentage of fruit
intake that comes
from juices
for children aged
two to five

Meat, Fish, Eggs,
Nuts and Beans

- Grilled chicken breast
- Sirloin steak
- Grilled salmon or tuna steak
- Lean turkey, ham, or beef slices
- Scrambled, poached, or boiled eggs
- Stewed kidney beans
- Hummus
- Natural, unsweetened peanut butter*

Dietary protein is the body's mechanic, repairing everything from cell walls to cuts to broken bones. It also drives metabolism, so increasing your child's lean protein consumption will make his or her body more efficient at burning calories. For meats, the most important factors are that the cuts and the cooking methods are naturally lean. That means grilling or roasting chicken, pork loin, and less-marbled cuts of beef like sirloin and fillet.

Perfect for fruit and veggie dipping. Check the ingredients list and opt for a natural peanut butter without sugar and partially hydrogenated oils.

Fruits

- Sliced apples or pears
- Berries (straight, or on yogurt or cereal)
- Bananas
- Grapes
- 100 percent fruit smoothies

So much of the fruit consumed by children is heavily processed; fruit is crushed to make juice or smashed into sweet snacks and bars. What you want is whole, unadulterated fruits in their most natural forms—even if that means buying them frozen. Actually, studies show that frozen fruit can be more nutrient packed because it's packaged during peak season. Taken together, fruits and vegetables should compose at least half of your child's daily dietary plate.

Dairy

- Semi-skimmed milk
- Cottage cheese
- Plain yogurt with fresh fruit

Dairy products are great sources of protein and bone-building calcium, but the high fat content means they can pack plenty of calories. On the flip side, going fat free means your child can lose out on some of the nutrients in dairy—a bit of fat will help your body absorb them properly. That's why we like low-fat dairy products such as semi-skimmed milk and reduced-fat cheese: They have enough fat to make them nutritious, but won't pack on the pounds.

Grains

- Brown rice
- Wholemeal bread
- Quinoa
- Wholemeal pasta
- Porridge

This list's superiority is partially due to its lower glycemic index (meaning that the carbohydrates have less of an impact on the blood sugar level) and the boost in protein provided by some of the foods (quinoa is the best). However, it's the fibre that matters most. Many of these grains cram in double what their non-wholemeal counterparts contain. For kids, starting this habit now will not only fend off diabetes, but also reduce the risk of cancer and heart disease later in life.

22

Percentage of bread consumed in the UK that is brown or wholemeal

Vegetables

- Steamed broccoli
- Mixed green salad
- Sautéed mushrooms
- Roasted squash
- Grilled sweet peppers and onions
- Baby carrots
- Sweet potatoes

Stick with raw vegetables or minimally cooked ones to retain the potent nutrients. And shop the rainbow. By choosing deep green, red, orange and white vegetables, you're guaranteed to consume a balance of vitamins and minerals. One easy-to-make switch is from white potatoes to the sweet version, which lowers the impact on blood sugar levels and makes you feel fuller for longer.

Meat, Poultry, Fish, Eggs, and Beans

- Chicken nuggets
- Fried chicken
- Fried battered cod
- High-fat processed sausages
- Burgers
- Fatty cuts of steak
- Peanut butter with added sugars and partially hydrogenated fats

An abnormally large percentage of kids' protein consumption is in the form of chicken nuggets. It doesn't take a genius to know that caked-on crumbs submerged in molten oil are a surefire way to increase their calorie intake. So is opting for fatty cuts of beef like mince (used to make burgers) and ribeye steaks (loaded with intramuscular fat).

7.3
Pounds gained over a year by eating one Big Mac's worth of calories more than you expend every week

23
The average number of ingredients (apart from chicken) in a fast food chicken nugget

Fruits

- More than 250ml of juice a day
- More than an adult handful of dried fruit a day
- Smoothies made with added sugar or cream
- Canned fruit in syrup

These choices might be better than a bag of Skittles, but not by much. Drinking your fruits in the form of juices or non-whole-fruit smoothies makes you miss out on one of fruits' biggest benefits—fibre. And fruit-flavoured packaged foods are just that: industrially processed items heavy with sugar and light in actual fruit. On the entire plate, whole foods are better than processed ones.

17
Teaspoons of added sugar most five-year-olds eat every single day

Not That!

Dairy
- Chocolate milk
- Ice cream
- Full-fat cheese sauces
- Yogurt with a high sugar content

Most people think about reducing the fat content of dairy, and that can be helpful, since many of the listed foods are chock-full of it. But equally as significant nowadays are the spoonfuls of sugar added to so many milk products. Just one serving of Nesquik Chocolate Milk contains over 21 grams of sugar—more than in a bag of Maltesers.

28
Percentage of vegetables eaten in chip form by children and teenagers

Grains
- White rice
- White bread
- Muffins
- Pancakes
- High-sugar cereals

Quick-burning carbohydrates, the kind found in these refined grains, take a child's blood sugar on a bumpy ride. And that has short-term and long-term consequences. Increased sugar consumption has been linked not just to weight gain and obesity, but also to hyperactivity, ADHD, anxiety and reduced school performance.

Vegetables
- Chips
- Crisps
- Onion rings
- White potatoes

Don't negate the benefits of vegetables by frying them. The deep-fryer treatment not only zaps vegetables of most of their nutrients, but also subjects them to oils loaded with excess calories and fat.

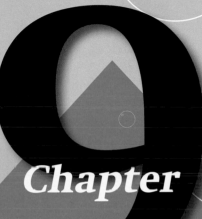

9
Chapter

WHAT ARE YOU DRINKING?

The Anatomy of your drink

Ever wonder what you're really drinking? The list of additives currently approved by the EU is staggeringly long. And no doubt more than a fair few can be found floating around in your favourite beverage. Find out how these 10 popular drinks are made—from the healthy and straightforward to the disturbingly scientific.

Cola

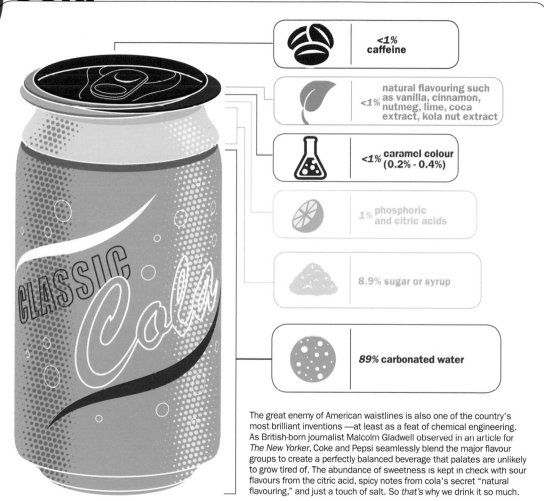

<1%
caffeine

<1% natural flavouring such as vanilla, cinnamon, nutmeg, lime, coca extract, kola nut extract

<1% **caramel colour** (0.2% - 0.4%)

1% phosphoric and citric acids

8.9% sugar or syrup

89% **carbonated water**

The great enemy of American waistlines is also one of the country's most brilliant inventions —at least as a feat of chemical engineering. As British-born journalist Malcolm Gladwell observed in an article for *The New Yorker*, Coke and Pepsi seamlessly blend the major flavour groups to create a perfectly balanced beverage that palates are unlikely to grow tired of. The abundance of sweetness is kept in check with sour flavours from the citric acid, spicy notes from cola's secret "natural flavouring," and just a touch of salt. So *that's* why we drink it so much.

Beer

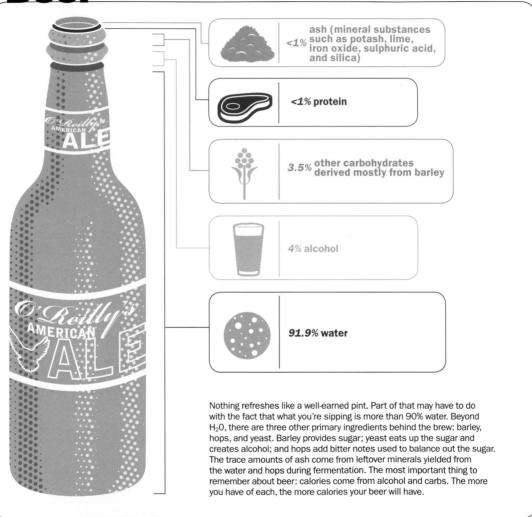

<1% ash (mineral substances such as potash, lime, iron oxide, sulphuric acid, and silica)

<1% protein

3.5% other carbohydrates derived mostly from barley

4% alcohol

91.9% water

Nothing refreshes like a well-earned pint. Part of that may have to do with the fact that what you're sipping is more than 90% water. Beyond H_2O, there are three other primary ingredients behind the brew: barley, hops, and yeast. Barley provides sugar; yeast eats up the sugar and creates alcohol; and hops add bitter notes used to balance out the sugar. The trace amounts of ash come from leftover minerals yielded from the water and hops during fermentation. The most important thing to remember about beer: calories come from alcohol and carbs. The more you have of each, the more calories your beer will have.

Coffee Drink

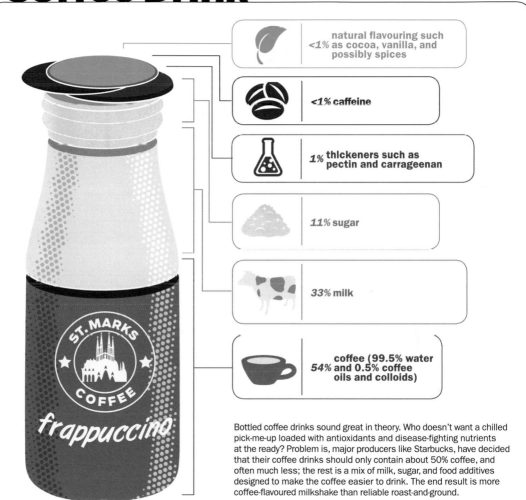

<1% natural flavouring such as cocoa, vanilla, and possibly spices

<1% caffeine

1% thickeners such as pectin and carrageenan

11% sugar

33% milk

54% coffee (99.5% water and 0.5% coffee oils and colloids)

ST. MARKS COFFEE

frappuccino

Bottled coffee drinks sound great in theory. Who doesn't want a chilled pick-me-up loaded with antioxidants and disease-fighting nutrients at the ready? Problem is, major producers like Starbucks, have decided that their coffee drinks should only contain about 50% coffee, and often much less; the rest is a mix of milk, sugar, and food additives designed to make the coffee easier to drink. The end result is more coffee-flavoured milkshake than reliable roast-and-ground.

Cranberry Juice Drink

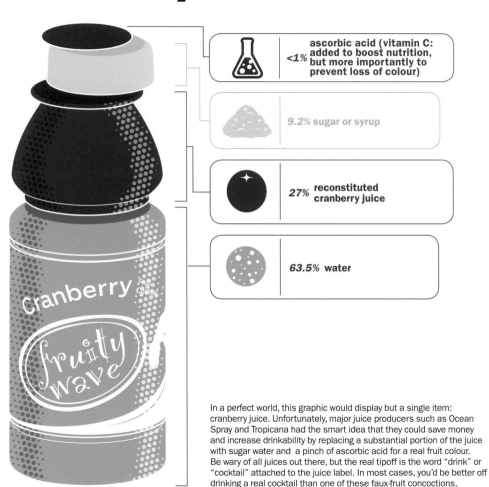

<1% ascorbic acid (vitamin C: added to boost nutrition, but more importantly to prevent loss of colour)

9.2% sugar or syrup

27% reconstituted cranberry juice

63.5% water

In a perfect world, this graphic would display but a single item: cranberry juice. Unfortunately, major juice producers such as Ocean Spray and Tropicana had the smart idea that they could save money and increase drinkability by replacing a substantial portion of the juice with sugar water and a pinch of ascorbic acid for a real fruit colour. Be wary of all juices out there, but the real tipoff is the word "drink" or "cocktail" attached to the juice label. In most cases, you'd be better off drinking a real cocktail than one of these faux-fruit concoctions.

Vegetable Juice

WHAT ARE YOU DRINKING?

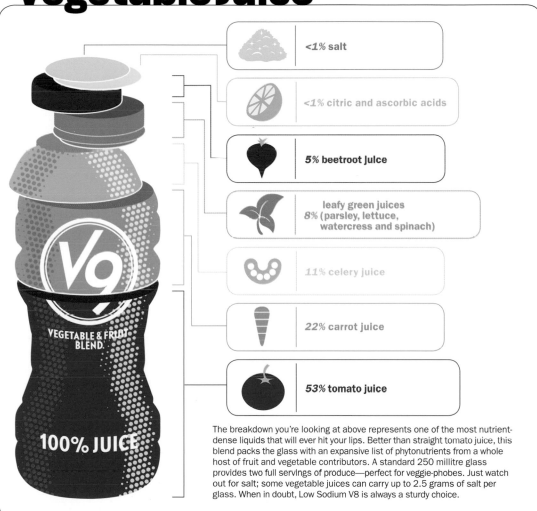

<1% salt

<1% citric and ascorbic acids

5% beetroot juice

8% leafy green juices (parsley, lettuce, watercress and spinach)

11% celery juice

22% carrot juice

53% tomato juice

The breakdown you're looking at above represents one of the most nutrient-dense liquids that will ever hit your lips. Better than straight tomato juice, this blend packs the glass with an expansive list of phytonutrients from a whole host of fruit and vegetable contributors. A standard 250 millilitre glass provides two full servings of produce—perfect for veggie-phobes. Just watch out for salt; some vegetable juices can carry up to 2.5 grams of salt per glass. When in doubt, Low Sodium V8 is always a sturdy choice.

Lemonade

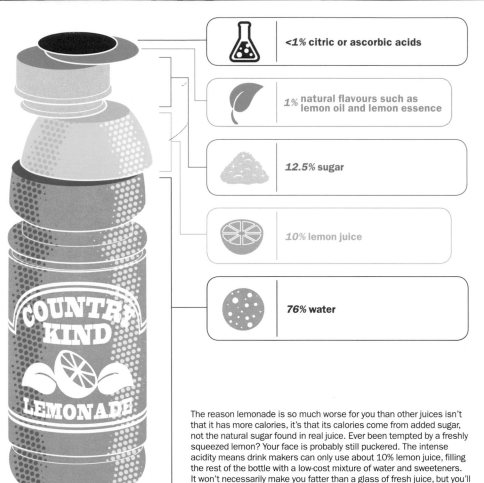

<1% citric or ascorbic acids

1% natural flavours such as lemon oil and lemon essence

12.5% sugar

10% lemon juice

76% water

The reason lemonade is so much worse for you than other juices isn't that it has more calories, it's that its calories come from added sugar, not the natural sugar found in real juice. Ever been tempted by a freshly squeezed lemon? Your face is probably still puckered. The intense acidity means drink makers can only use about 10% lemon juice, filling the rest of the bottle with a low-cost mixture of water and sweeteners. It won't necessarily make you fatter than a glass of fresh juice, but you'll miss out on the nutritional punch found in that other 90% of real fruit.

Energy Drink

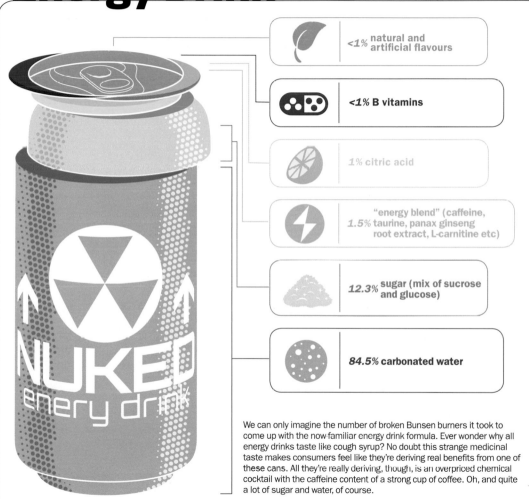

<1% natural and artificial flavours

<1% B vitamins

1% citric acid

1.5% "energy blend" (caffeine, taurine, panax ginseng root extract, L-carnitine etc)

12.3% sugar (mix of sucrose and glucose)

84.5% carbonated water

NUKED
enery drink

We can only imagine the number of broken Bunsen burners it took to come up with the now-familiar energy drink formula. Ever wonder why all energy drinks taste like cough syrup? No doubt this strange medicinal taste makes consumers feel like they're deriving real benefits from one of these cans. All they're really deriving, though, is an overpriced chemical cocktail with the caffeine content of a strong cup of coffee. Oh, and quite a lot of sugar and water, of course.

Vitamin-Enhanced Water

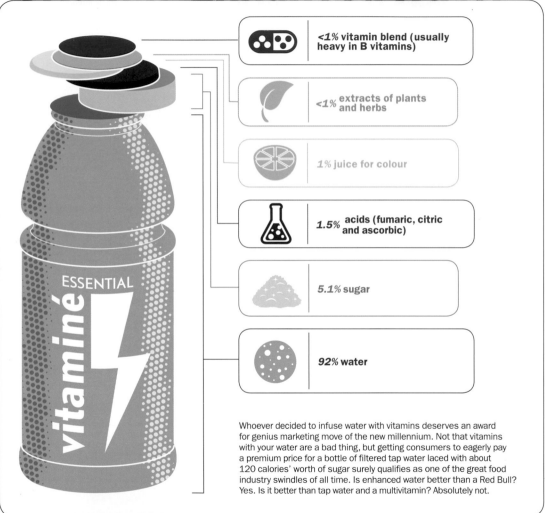

<1% vitamin blend (usually heavy in B vitamins)

<1% extracts of plants and herbs

1% juice for colour

1.5% acids (fumaric, citric and ascorbic)

5.1% sugar

92% water

ESSENTIAL

vitaminé

Whoever decided to infuse water with vitamins deserves an award for genius marketing move of the new millennium. Not that vitamins with your water are a bad thing, but getting consumers to eagerly pay a premium price for a bottle of filtered tap water laced with about 120 calories' worth of sugar surely qualifies as one of the great food industry swindles of all time. Is enhanced water better than a Red Bull? Yes. Is it better than tap water and a multivitamin? Absolutely not.

Chocolate Milk

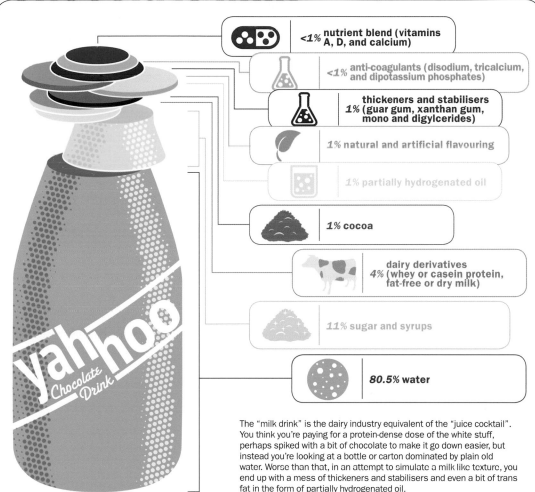

<1% nutrient blend (vitamins A, D, and calcium)

<1% anti-coagulants (disodium, tricalcium, and dipotassium phosphates)

1% thickeners and stabilisers (guar gum, xanthan gum, mono and digylcerides)

1% natural and artificial flavouring

1% partially hydrogenated oil

1% cocoa

4% dairy derivatives (whey or casein protein, fat-free or dry milk)

11% sugar and syrups

80.5% water

The "milk drink" is the dairy industry equivalent of the "juice cocktail". You think you're paying for a protein-dense dose of the white stuff, perhaps spiked with a bit of chocolate to make it go down easier, but instead you're looking at a bottle or carton dominated by plain old water. Worse than that, in an attempt to simulate a milk like texture, you end up with a mess of thickeners and stabilisers and even a bit of trans fat in the form of partially hydrogenated oil.

Index

Boldface page references indicate photographs with text.

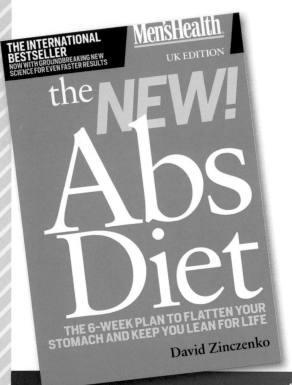